CONTENTS

STATEMENTS

THURSDAY, OCTOBER 24, 2002

ADDITIONAL MATERIAL

S. Hrg. 107–747

UNINSURED PREGNANT WOMEN: IMPACT ON INFANT AND MATERNAL MORTALITY

HEARING

BEFORE THE

SUBCOMMITTEE ON PUBLIC HEALTH

OF THE

COMMITTEE ON HEALTH, EDUCATION, LABOR, AND PENSIONS
UNITED STATES SENATE

ONE HUNDRED SEVENTH CONGRESS

SECOND SESSION

ON

EXAMINING THE IMPACT OF UNINSURED PREGNANT WOMEN ON INFANT AND MATERNAL MORTALITY

OCTOBER 24, 2002

Printed for the use of the Committee on Health, Education, Labor, and Pensions

U.S. GOVERNMENT PRINTING OFFICE

82–564 PDF WASHINGTON : 2003

For sale by the Superintendent of Documents, U.S. Government Printing Office
Internet: bookstore.gpo.gov Phone: toll free (866) 512–1800; DC area (202) 512–1800
Fax: (202) 512–2250 Mail: Stop SSOP, Washington, DC 20402–0001

COMMITTEE ON HEALTH, EDUCATION, LABOR, AND PENSIONS

EDWARD M. KENNEDY, Massachusetts, *Chairman*

CHRISTOPHER J. DODD, Connecticut
TOM HARKIN, Iowa
BARBARA A. MIKULSKI, Maryland
JAMES M. JEFFORDS (I), Vermont
JEFF BINGAMAN, New Mexico
PAUL D. WELLSTONE, Minnesota
PATTY MURRAY, Washington
JACK REED, Rhode Island
JOHN EDWARDS, North Carolina
HILLARY RODHAM CLINTON, New York

JUDD GREGG, New Hampshire
BILL FRIST, Tennessee
MICHAEL B. ENZI, Wyoming
TIM HUTCHINSON, Arkansas
JOHN W. WARNER, Virginia
CHRISTOPHER S. BOND, Missouri
PAT ROBERTS, Kansas
SUSAN M. COLLINS, Maine
JEFF SESSIONS, Alabama
MIKE DeWINE, Ohio

J. MICHAEL MYERS, *Staff Director and Chief Counsel*
TOWNSEND LANGE MCNITT, *Minority Staff Director*

SUBCOMMITTEE ON PUBLIC HEALTH

EDWARD M. KENNEDY, *Chairman*

TOM HARKIN, Iowa
BARBARA A. MIKULSKI, Maryland
JAMES M. JEFFORDS, Vermont
JEFF BINGAMAN, New Mexico
PAUL D. WELLSTONE, Minnesota
JACK REED, Rhode Island
JOHN EDWARDS, North Carolina
HILLARY RODHAM CLINTON, New York

BILL FRIST, Tennessee
JUDD GREGG, New Hampshire
MICHAEL B. ENZI, Wyoming
TIM HUTCHINSON, Arkansas
PAT ROBERTS, Kansas
SUSAN M. COLLINS, Maine
JEFF SESSIONS, Alabama
CHRISTOPHER S. BOND, Missouri

DAVID NEXON, *Staff Director*
DEAN A. ROSEN, *Minority Staff Director*

UNINSURED PREGNANT WOMEN: IMPACT ON INFANT AND MATERNAL MORTALITY

THURSDAY, OCTOBER 24, 2002

U.S. SENATE,
SUBCOMMITTEE ON PUBLIC HEALTH,
OF THE COMMITTEE ON HEALTH, EDUCATION, LABOR, AND PENSIONS,
Washington, DC.

The subcommittee met, pursuant to notice, at 10:07 a.m., in room SD–430, Dirksen Senate Office Building, Senator Bingaman presiding.

Present: Senator Bingaman.

OPENING STATEMENT OF SENATOR BINGAMAN

Senator BINGAMAN. Why don't we go ahead and get started? Thank you all for being here.

First I would like to thank Senator Kennedy for allowing us to hold this important hearing with respect to the health and well-being both of children and their mothers.

Our Nation ranks 28th in the world in infant mortality and 21st in maternal mortality, according to the data from the CDC. In infant mortality, for example, our country ranks behind Spain and Portugal, the Czech Republic and Cuba. There are numerous studies that have shown the importance of providing coverage to pregnant women in order to reduce both infant and maternal mortality. We, as a Nation, would be remiss to not take the simple but critical step of increasing access to prenatal and labor and delivery and postpartum care through the State Children's Health Insurance Program or SCHIP to help prevent birth defects and prematurity, the most common causes of infant death and disability, as well as maternal death and disability.

It is with this in mind that a number of bills were introduced in this Congress to address these problems by allowing states the option to expand health coverage to uninsured pregnant women over the age of 18 through the State Children's Health Insurance Program or SCHIP. Those bills include S. 724, the Mothers and Newborns Health Insurance Act that Senators Bond and Breaux introduced. Senator Lincoln and I are cosponsors on that. I think Senator Corzine is, as well. He is just entering at this moment. There is also S. 1016, the Start Healthy, Stay Healthy Act, which again Senator Lugar, Senator Lincoln, Senator Corzine, Senator McCain and I all cosponsored and there is S. 1244, the Family Care Act that Senators Kennedy and Snowe introduced. All of these try to address this issue of increasing access to care for pregnant women.

Throughout the early part of the year the Secretary of Health and Human Services, Secretary Thompson, issued press releases and testified before Congress, wrote letters in support of the passage of legislation to cover pregnant women. He wrote me on the 12th of April of this year and that letter said, "The prenatal care for women and their babies is a crucial part of medical care. These services can be a vital life-long determinant of health and we should do everything we can to make this care available for all pregnant women. It is one of the most important investments we can make for the long-term good health of our Nation. As I testified recently at a hearing by the Health Subcommittee of the House Energy and Commerce Committee, I also support legislation to expand SCHIP to cover pregnant women. However, because legislation has not moved and because of the importance of prenatal care, I felt it important to take this action."

Now this action that he is referring to was the issuance of a regulation to allow the coverage of unborn through SCHIP. The rule which was initially proposed this past spring and issued in final form on the 2nd of October, allows states the option to cover unborn children through SCHIP but not to cover pregnant women. It came just 2 weeks after Deputy Assistant Secretary Cristina Beato testified at a hearing here in this room on Hispanic health that the administration would be forthcoming with a letter in support of S. 724 and also 1 week after the administration approved a waiver for the State of Colorado to cover pregnant women through the SCHIP program.

Colorado clearly faced the choice of taking the State option of covering unborn children as a result of the new regulation or the alternative that was more cumbersome and the more lengthy process of applying for a waiver to cover pregnant women. According to State officials, Colorado chose the more cumbersome waiver process because they were unable to implement coverage for unborn children. There is no insurance program anywhere on which to model that coverage. There were too many questions that they could not answer. They were also concerned by the gaps in coverage for pregnant women that the regulation caused.

Among other things, since the regulation only provides states the option to cover unborn children, a number of important aspects of coverage for pregnant women during all states of birth—pregnancy, labor and delivery and postpartum care—are either denied or in serious question. For example, pregnant women would likely not be covered during their pregnancy for treatment of some kinds of cancer, medical emergencies, accidents, broken bones or mental illness. Even life-saving surgery for a mother in certain circumstances would appear to be denied.

Further, during delivery, coverage for an epidural would be a State option and allowed only if the health of the child is judged to be affected. On the other hand, anesthesia is covered for Caesarian sections, so the rule could wrongly push women and providers to perform unnecessary C-sections to ensure coverage of critical pain relief for pregnant women.

Finally, during the postpartum period women would be denied all health care coverage from the moment the child is born. As the regulation reads, “Commenters are correct that care after delivery, such as postpartum services, could not be covered as part of SCHIP because they are not services for an eligible child.” Important care and treatment, including but not limited to treatment of hemorrhage, infection, pregnancy-induced hypertension and other complications of pregnancy and childbirth, including life-saving treatment, would not be covered.

In contrast, the legislation that we have been proposing explicitly covers the full range of pregnancy-related services, including postpartum care. This is important as the majority of maternal deaths occur in the postpartum period and should be covered.

The legislation is also, of course, about improving children’s health. We all know the importance of an infant’s first year of life. Senator Bond’s legislation, as amended in the Finance Committee with language from the bill that I had earlier introduced, provides 12 months of continuous coverage for children after birth. In contrast, the administration regulation provides 12 months’ continuous enrollment to states but makes the time retroactive to cover the period in the womb. Therefore, if nine full months of prenatal care are provided, the child could lose coverage after 3 months following the child’s birth. This obviously would make it difficult to have coverage for well-baby visits, immunizations and access to a pediatric caregiver during the first year of life.

Senators Bond and Lincoln and I tried both on October 2 and then again Senator Corzine and Landrieu joined us on October 8; we tried to get consent to pass S. 724, the Mothers and Newborns Health Insurance Act. This was passed out of the Finance Committee without opposition in July. Unfortunately, on both occasions our Republicans colleagues objected, citing the opposition of the administration.

To our surprise, Secretary Thompson had reversed his position and issued a letter to Senator Nichols on October 8 dropping his support for passage of the legislation by saying that, in his view, “The regulation is a more effective and comprehensive solution to the issue.” This reversal came despite the fact that there are, in my view, at least, glaring gaps in the administration’s regulation that are acknowledged in the rule itself.

Let me at this point just indicate that the administration was invited to testify by Senator Gregg’s office and Senator Kennedy’s office, declined to do so on the basis they had not been given adequate notice of the hearing. We respect that position. I very much hope that they will submit written testimony for us to include in the record, as many other groups and parties have indicated they intend to.

[The prepared statement of Senator Kennedy follows:]

Prepared Statement of Senator Kennedy

One of the most serious aspects of the health care crisis that continues to affect so many of our fellow citizens is the lack of access by large numbers of pregnant women to affordable health care. Excellent prenatal care is available in this country, but 14 percent of pregnant women today do not have the opportunity to benefit from it and over 11 million more women of child bearing age are at risk of not having such care because they are uninsured. The lack of prenatal care for these women can lead to illness and loss of life.

In fact, the United States ranks 21st in the world in infant mortality and 26th in maternal mortality the highest rates of any developed nation. These mortality statistics are unacceptable, and it is even more frustrating is that these deaths are largely preventable.

We know that timely prenatal care leads to positive health outcomes for mothers and newborns. Such care assures that pregnant women receive guidance on proper nutrition and encourages the elimination of unhealthy habits such as drinking and smoking. It also prevents transmission of disease from mother to fetus, and helps to avoid pregnancy-related complications.

CDC has released data indicating that routine screening for group B strep in late pregnancy is the most effective way to prevent its transmission from mother to child during pregnancy. Screening for diabetes can prevent complications during pregnancy and birth. Prenatal care can also prevent transmission of Hepatitis B and HIV from mother to child. These are all simple steps that can prevent illness and death if women have access to good health care. Insurance coverage will give pregnant women access to the care they need to be healthy before and after birth, and give infants a chance for a truly healthy start in life.

Many Senators have introduced legislation to provide access to prenatal care services. Senator Bingaman has proposed legislation to assure that pregnant women receive effective care during pregnancy and after birth, and I commend him for his leadership on this important issue. Senator Harkin and Senator Snowe are also leaders on this issue, and I commend them as well. We need to do all we can in Congress to end this key aspect of the nation's health crisis.

When we provide mothers and their children with access to good health care, we are investing wisely in the future of our country.

Senator BINGAMAN. Let me go ahead with our first panel of witnesses here. We are very fortunate to have Senators Lincoln and Corzine. Let me just give a very brief introduction to both of them. They have both been real champions on this issue since the beginning. Senator Lincoln, as she stated on the Senate floor a couple of times, is not only a champion of the bill but an expert on the subject. She is one of the Senate's leading advocates on the issues of children and women's health. She had one of the very first pieces of legislation to expand coverage to pregnant women in the previous Congress, legislation entitled "The Improved Maternal and Children's Health Act of 2000." In this Congress she has been a supporter of both S. 724 and S. 1016, a cosponsor of both, and successfully helped push for the passage of S. 724 out of the Senate Finance Committee in July.

Senator Corzine has been a strong champion of this legislation, as well. He was an original cosponsor of S. 1016. He has worked closely with me at every stage of getting this legislation passed. He has taken the next step of putting his interest into direct action in New Jersey and is working with the What to Expect Foundation on helping low-income mothers receive prenatal care and literacy education to improve their pregnancies and subsequent parenthood. Based on that work, we have begun to initiate a similar program in New Mexico and I want to thank him and Lisa Bernstein both, who will be testifying on the second panel, for their dedication and testimony today on this important issue.

Let me call on Senator Lincoln first and then Senator Corzine on any comments they have and then we will move to our second panel.

STATEMENTS OF HON. JON CORZINE, A U.S. SENATOR FROM THE STATE OF NEW JERSEY; AND HON. BLANCHE LINCOLN, A U.S. SENATOR FROM THE STATE OF ARKANSAS

Senator LINCOLN. Mr. Chairman, I am going to allow my colleague to have a few comments, as he has got to run to the floor and open the Senate. So I am going to defer to him.

Senator BINGAMAN. Senator Corzine, we are glad to hear from you first.

Senator CORZINE. I appreciate Senator Lincoln yielding. I have about a 10-minute open in the Senate and then put us into recess. So I apologize that I have to leave and come back and I will join you.

I congratulate you, Mr. Chairman, for your efforts on this very important subject, and Senator Lincoln and others, because it is one that we are not giving the right attention to and I join your comments.

Senator BINGAMAN. Thank you very much. And when you return I obviously invite you and Senator Lincoln to participate here in the rest of the hearing on the panel.

Senator Lincoln, go right ahead.

Senator LINCOLN. Thank you, Mr. Chairman. Certainly a particularly overwhelming thank you to you, Chairman Bingaman, for allowing me to participate today and for making this hearing happen. Your dedication to women and children's health is absolutely exceptional. As a mother and as a senator, I am proud of the leadership that you have demonstrated time and again on this very important issue.

As you know, the Senate currently has the historic opportunity to enact legislation, the Mothers and Newborns Health Insurance Act, S. 724, which you have commented on, that could drastically improve the lives and health of thousands of women and children throughout our Nation. This bipartisan legislation, which we both cosponsored and helped to pass unanimously in the Finance Committee this summer, gives states the option, simply the option, of covering pregnant women in their Children's Health Insurance Programs. Most importantly, the bill allows coverage for prenatal care, delivery and postpartum care.

Mr. Chairman, the statistics you have often cited about infant and maternal mortality in this great country of ours are absolutely inexcusable. According to the Centers for Disease Control and Prevention, the U.S. ranks 28th in the world in infant mortality. We rank behind countries like Cuba and the Czech Republic. It is amazing to me that the United States lags far behind these nations in this area.

Another shocking statistic from the CDC is that the U.S. ranks 21st in the world in maternal mortality. The World Health Organization estimates that the United States maternal mortality rate is double that of Canada.

The chart right here that I have brought to share with you all today, the graph shows the data from the CDC on maternal mortality in the U.S. from 1967 to 1999. The data shows that the rate of maternal mortality has dramatically decreased since the' 60s but this decrease has leveled off, and you can see as it begins to flatline down there.

In 1999 there were 8.3 maternal deaths per 100,000 lives births in the U.S., far above the CDC's Healthy People 2000 goal of 3.3 maternal deaths. In fact, you can see on the graph that the maternal death rates have been steady or rising since the mid-1980s. This means that since 1983 the United States has made no progress in achieving its own goal of a 3.3 maternal death rate.

Even more upsetting is that in the United States an African-American woman's risk of dying from pregnancy or pregnancy-related complications is four times greater than the risk faced by white women. This is one of the largest racial disparities among public health indicators and one that we really see in Arkansas, where the maternal mortality rate for African-American women is 12.4. That is 66 percent higher than the national maternal mortality rate.

I am absolutely ashamed of these statistics. When we are ahead of every other Nation in almost every other arena I am ashamed we have not taken a course of action that would prove to the rest of the world that we truly do value life in this country and that we want to do all we possibly can to ensure the healthy delivery of children, as well as the health of their mothers.

The fact is we know how to address this problem. The solution lies in prenatal and postpartum care. Studies have shown that this care significantly reduces infant mortality, maternal mortality, and the number of low birth weight babies, not to mention the quality of life of these individuals later on.

Not only is prenatal care essential for quality of life; it is also cost-effective. For every dollar we spend on prenatal care we save more than $6 in neonatal intensive care costs, not to mention the cost to the woman who is giving birth. Preterm births are one of the most expensive reasons for a hospital stay in the United States, not to mention the difficulties these children have later in life, whether it is learning disabilities or health care issues and complications. There are a number of things that give us reason why it is so important to make this investment in prenatal care.

I cannot emphasize enough the great opportunity that we have here in the Senate to drastically improve the lives and the health of women and babies in our country. We must pass S. 724 as soon as possible. The states want to cover pregnant women under SCHIP and the Federal Government should give them the option.

Mr. Chairman, I was proud to join you and Senator Bond on the Senate floor in recent weeks to try and bring up and pass S. 724 and I am so frustrated that both our attempts to pass this bill were blocked. It is a shame that some of our colleagues have made a political issue out of trying to ensure a healthy start in life for babies and their mothers.

I am disappointed that Secretary Thompson has recently withdrawn his support for S. 724 in favor of the administration's final regulation to provide SCHIP coverage to unborn children. I do know what it is that has all of a sudden crossed his mind to change his mind about the effectiveness of the legislation that we have presented back earlier this year.

All of this concerns me because the regulation fails to cover the full scope of medical services needed by a woman during and after pregnancy that are recommended by the American College of Obstetricians and Gynecologists and the American Academy of Pediatricians. We are not just saying this because some of us have been through it. We are not just saying it because our constituents think it is important or that they want it. We are saying it because medicine and science tells us how important this is.

I am certainly glad that representatives from these groups are here today to better explain these clinical standards of care and why they are critical to improving maternal and child health.

Many things concern me about the administration's regulation, Mr. Chairman. First, the regulation specifically states that postpartum care is not covered. Postpartum care is essential in treating serious pregnancy-related complications for the new mother, complications that can often lead to death. Where does that leave a newborn child?

According to the National Committee for Quality Assurance, hemorrhage, pregnancy-induced hypertension, infection and ectopic pregnancy continue to account for more than half of all maternal deaths. Why would we not want to guarantee insurance coverage for postpartum care to ensure that women will receive proper treatment for these complications? Consider our country's efforts to reduce maternal mortality rates. The regulation's silence on this issue is extremely disturbing.

Postpartum care is covered by Medicaid and most private insurance. What if the new mother has a hemorrhage, an infection, she needs an episiotomy repaired or has postpartum depression? The administration's regulation would not cover such services because in their words, they are not services for an eligible child.

Given this huge gap in coverage and the political complications of this regulation, I am worried that states will ignore it and continue to try to provide coverage to pregnant women through the HHS waiver process, which many states have already done. But governors and State legislators have argued that this waiver process is lengthy and cumbersome. They prefer a State option that is easier to administer and that is permanent. That is why they support S. 724.

The regulation also causes me to wonder about provider reimbursement. Under the regulation, doctors will not be reimbursed for providing care that they have been trained to provide and likely feel that they are ethically obligated to provide. In the modern practice of obstetrics, postpartum care is a critical part of the treatment the woman receives prenatally and during labor and delivery. With rising medical malpractice rates, particularly for obstetricians and gynecologists, these doctors may simply decide to stop serving

SCHIP patients. This regulation may become yet another disincentive for doctors to participate in public programs serving low-income populations.

Finally, I must say as a woman I am offended by the administration's regulation. How they can leave the woman totally out of the equation when talking about pregnancy is beyond me, Mr. Chairman. Women's bodies change and they grow during the pregnancy. Her psyche may change, too. Many of you husbands have witnessed that and believe me, it is not easy.

S. 724, on the other hand, puts mother and baby on equal footing by guaranteeing that they both have access to the recommended clinical care that they both need.

Having given birth to twins 6 years ago, I can personally attest to the importance of prenatal and postpartum care. Because I had this care, I was blessed with two healthy boys and a relatively trouble-free pregnancy and delivery. Both boys and I were able to come home from the hospital within 2 days to a healthy beginning for our entire family. I was able to nurse my children with the guidance of my physicians and the guidance that I could get in my postpartum care. No one should stand in the way of encouraging healthy pregnancies for the most vulnerable women in our country.

On behalf of our Nation's mothers, fathers and their babies, we in the Senate have the serious obligation to pass this legislation as soon as possible. If we truly value life, as we say we do, we will take action on something that will provide us and those families the ability to do all that they possibly can to ensure a healthy delivery and a healthy start for these children.

Let us come together in a bipartisan way and pass S. 724, legislation that will make a difference not only in a child's life, a woman's life, a family's life, but certainly, Mr. Chairman, in our Nation's success.

I thank you again, Mr. Chairman, for holding this hearing and certainly for your leadership in this arena. I look forward to hearing the testimony today that will likely underscore the need for passing S. 724 as soon as possible. And on behalf of the women and children and families out there, I do encourage us all not to let this become a political issue but more importantly, to recognize its importance. Thank you, Mr. Chairman.

Senator BINGAMAN. Thank you very much for your very strong statement. Why do you not join us up here if your schedule permits? We are anxious to have you participate in the question and answer part of this.

Senator Bond is the prime sponsor on the legislation and, as Senator Lincoln has pointed out very eloquently, it is bipartisan. We have strong support from many of our Republican colleagues for moving ahead with this bill, S. 724, and we hope that we are able to do that when we come back into session.

If all the witnesses would come forward, let me introduce all of the witnesses in a group here and then we will just call on them to testify.

Dr. Nancy Green is with the March of Dimes Foundation. Dr. Green is a pediatrician and the medical director for the March of Dimes Foundation in White Plains, NY. Dr. Green also serves as associate professor of pediatrics and cell biology at the Albert Einstein College of Medicine, is a leading national expert on topics in pediatric hematology, oncology, immunology and genetics.

Dr. Laura Riley is with Massachusetts General. She is here on behalf of the American College of Obstetricians and Gynecologists. Dr. Riley is a nationally recognized expert on the delivery and care for at-risk pregnant women and is testifying today on behalf of this American College of Obstetricians and Gynecologists. She is the medical director of labor and delivery at Mass General Hospital in Boston, is the current chair of the Obstetrics Practice Committee at the American College of Obstetricians and Gynecologists.

Dr. Richard Bucciarelli is with the University of Florida Department of Pediatrics and is here on behalf of the American Academy of Pediatrics. He is a long-time authority and advocate for the American Academy of Pediatrics for the betterment of children's health. He is a nationwide expert on improving health coverage and quality of care for children with special health care needs. He is currently a professor and associate chairman in the Department of Pediatrics at the University of Florida College of Medicine and a professor at the Institute for Child Health Policy in Gainesville, FL.

And Lisa Bernstein is with the What to Expect Foundation. She is co-founder and executive director of that foundation in New York City. The foundation takes its name from the best-selling What to Expect pregnancy and parenting series that was co-written by the foundation's president, Heidi Murkoff. The What to Expect series has been described by women across America as their pregnancy bible. The What to Expect Foundation is a nonprofit organization dedicated to assisting low-income women also to share in the knowledge and understanding of how to have healthy pregnancies and safe outcomes for themselves and their children through the Baby Basics program, which provides prenatal education to low-income women.

We have, as you can see from these introductions, a very distinguished set of witnesses. Dr. Green, why do you not start? We are eager to hear your testimony.

STATEMENTS OF NANCY GREEN, M.D., MEDICAL DIRECTOR, MARCH OF DIMES BIRTH DEFECTS FOUNDATION; RICHARD BUCCIARELLI, M.D., CHAIRMAN, AMERICAN ACADEMY OF PEDIATRICS SUBCOMMITTEE ON ACCESS TO HEALTH CARE; LISA BERNSTEIN, EXECUTIVE DIRECTOR, THE WHAT TO EXPECT FOUNDATION, NEW YORK, NY; AND LAURA E. RILEY, M.D., ASSISTANT PROFESSOR OF OB/GYN, HARVARD MEDICAL SCHOOL AND MEDICAL DIRECTOR OF LABOR AND DELIVERY, MASSACHUSETTS GENERAL HOSPITAL

Dr. GREEN. Thank you, Mr. Chairman. Good morning

I am Dr. Nancy Green. I am the medical director at the March of Dimes Birth Defects Foundation. The mission of the March of Dimes is to improve the health of babies by preventing birth defects and infant mortality, so this is an issue that is near and dear to our hearts.

I am pleased to be here today to discuss with you the importance of providing all pregnant women access to health insurance coverage and therefore access to a comprehensive set of basic maternity services. Lack of health coverage continues to be a significant problem for many Americans. Particularly troubling are the statistics on women of child-bearing age. 11.5 million women or nearly one in five women of child-bearing age went without health insurance in 2001, a higher rate than for other Americans under age 65. That means that some 28 percent of uninsured Americans are women of child-bearing age and several of you know that that lack of coverage is not equally distributed across our country. Women of Hispanic origin, Native Americans, African-Americans are disproportionately affected by this lack of health insurance.

Numerous studies have shown that having health insurance coverage affects how people use health care services. In a report issued earlier this year by the Institute of Medicine, researchers concluded that, and I quote, "Like Americans in general, pregnant women's use of health services varies by insurance status. Uninsured women receive fewer prenatal care services than their insured counterparts and report greater difficulty in obtaining the care that they believe they need."

We know how important prenatal care can be. In its report on pending legislation, the Senate Finance Committee stated that, "Recent studies have shown that infants born to mothers receiving late or no prenatal care are more likely to face complications which can result in hospitalization, expensive medical treatments, and increased cost to public programs. Closing the gap in coverage between mothers and their children will improve the health of both while reducing costs for taxpayers."

At the March of Dimes our overarching goal is to improve the health of mothers and their children. To further this goal, the foundation has worked throughout this Congress to obtain support for a modest incremental step to improve access to health service for uninsured pregnant women by amending the SCHIP program.

Mr. Chairman, S. 724, which includes provisions from your bill, S. 1016, the Healthy Start, Stay Healthy Act, would bring the SCHIP program into alignment with every other Federal health insurance program, all of which extend coverage to pregnant women and their babies. The provisions of S. 724 that are particularly important to advancing the mission of the March of Dimes include number one, allowing states the flexibility to extend SCHIP coverage to pregnant women 19 years and older and number two, automatically enrolling their newborns in the program and providing them with coverage for 12 months following birth.

Mr. Chairman, on several occasions throughout the year we were pleased that HHS Secretary Thompson endorsed legislation to achieve these important objectives. However, the March of Dimes is disappointed to learn that the administration has apparently withdrawn its support for legislation and instead will rely on a regulation that permits states to cover unborn children.

We are deeply concerned that this regulation fails to provide the mother the standard scope of maternity care services recommended here today by my colleagues at the American College of Obstetricians and Gynecologists and the American Academy of Pediatrics. Of particular concern, the regulation explicitly states that postpartum care is not covered. When a new mother goes home following delivery the March of Dimes wants to be sure that she is healthy enough to support herself, to breast-feed, to care for her newborn, and to participate in her family's life.

S. 724 has broad bipartisan support and the National Governors Association has called on Congress to give states this option. In addition, 26 national organizations have endorsed this initiative.

In short, S. 724 would give us and other organizations committed to improving the health of women and children the opportunity to work in states across the country to expand access to comprehensive basic maternity services, as recommended by obstetricians and pediatricians.

On behalf of the March of Dimes, thank you for your commitment to improving the health of children and their families and for this opportunity to testify on the issues of critical importance to pregnant women and infants.

Senator BINGAMAN. Thank you very much.

[The prepared statement of Dr. Green may be found in additional material.]

Senator BINGAMAN. Why do we not just go right down the table here? I think that is probably just as logical as anything else.

Dr. Bucciarelli, why do you not go right ahead?

Dr. BUCCIARELLI. Thank you, Mr. Chairman. Mr. Chairman, members of the committee, I am Richard Bucciarelli, a practicing neonatologist at the University of Florida, testifying today on behalf of the American Academy of Pediatrics.

As a practicing neonatologist, I am the physician that often takes care of the babies that are born too small, too sick to sometimes survive or even live up to their full potential. I am a former chairman of the American Academy of Pediatrics Committee on Federal Government Affairs and serve as the chairman of the Academy's Subcommittee on Access to Health Care. And on behalf of the Academy, I would like to thank the committee for the opportunity to present this statement.

Mr. Chairman, the Academy commends you and your colleagues and thank you for your leadership and determined efforts to dramatically reduce the number of uninsured children and pregnant women in this country. We look forward to actively working with you to bring health care coverage to all of our Nation's children and pregnant women.

The American Academy of Pediatrics is an organization of 57,000 pediatricians dedicated to the health, safety and well-being of infants, children, adolescents and young adults. A key principle for the Academy is that all children and pregnant women have the right to access age-appropriate quality health care.

Toward that end, the Academy is pleased to testify today in support of the Mothers and Newborns Health Insurance Act of 2002, S. 724. This legislation would give states the option of covering pregnant women with their State Children's Health Insurance Program and very importantly, it appropriates the additional funds to states to provide these necessary services. The Academy believes it is critically important that pregnant women receive the full range of medical services needed during their pregnancy and the postpartum period. These services are spelled out in the Guidelines for Prenatal Care, Fifth Edition, which was developed jointly by the American Academy of Pediatrics and the American College of

Obstetricians and Gynecologists. These guidelines describe the components of prenatal care that are needed by both the fetus and the pregnant woman to ensure early identification of risk factors and appropriate treatment of maternal fetal conditions.

As we all know, the administration published a final rule expanding SCHIP coverage to unborn children. The Academy is concerned that as written, this regulation falls dangerously short of the clinical standards of care outlined in our guidelines, which describe the importance of all stages of a birth—the pregnancy, delivery, and postpartum care. The Mothers and Newborns Health Insurance Act ensures that pregnant women can receive the critically important full range of prenatal and postpartum care.

This legislation, unlike the recently published rule, recognizes the important impact of the mother's health on the fetus. There is no doubt, for example, that maternal diabetes can directly affect the fetus and lead to increased mortality and morbidity and would be covered. But what about a mother with asthma in need of coverage to pay for her medications? Denial of coverage could result in a severe asthmatic attack, pneumonia, and could deprive the fetus of oxygen and lead to even premature delivery.

Or what about the mother with a severe infection of the gums of the mouth, gingivitis, and dental caries? How is this related to the fetus? Well, there is an increasing amount of data to indicate that chronic infection of the gums and bad dental health greatly increase the chances of a premature delivery with its increased morbidity, mortality and cost. And these are just two examples that demonstrate the importance of covering both the fetus and the pregnant woman with appropriate health benefits.

One of our biggest challenges we face as a Nation, and we have an opportunity to address that here today, is reducing the number of uninsured children and pregnant women in the United States. We believe the Mothers and Newborns Health Insurance Act takes an important step to decrease the number of uninsured children by providing 12 months of continuous eligibility for those children born to mothers under this act. It has been demonstrated that intermittent coverage compromises continuity of care, delays necessary therapy, and adds administrative costs for outreach and reenrollment efforts.

Additionally, this provision prevents newborns eligible for SCHIP from being subject to enrolment waiting periods, ensuring that infants receive appropriate health care in their first year of life. This legislation ensures that children born to women already enrolled in Medicaid or SCHIP are immediately enrolled in the program for which they are eligible. These provisions would provide presumptive and continuous eligibility for children covered under the act, guaranteeing essential uninterrupted access to health care throughout their first year of life, for it is within that first year of life when parents need the most assistance in dealing with their new child. It is within that first year of life that immunizations, timely immunizations, are most critical. And it is within that first year of life that making the correct diagnosis and initiating the appropriate therapy is so important.

We must make health care for America's children and pregnant women available, accessible and affordable. Providing children, adolescents and pregnant women access to quality care with an emphasis on prevention is truly an investment in our Nation's future. Thank you very much.

Senator BINGAMAN. Well, thank you very much.

Ms. Bernstein, why do you not go right ahead?

Ms. BERNSTEIN. Mr. Chairman, members of the committee, I am honored to come before you today to urge passage of S. 724, the Mothers and Newborns Health Insurance Act of 2001.

First, let me just tell you a bit of how I have come to be here and why the What to Expect Foundation was formed. The What to Expect Foundation takes its name, as you have heard, from the best-selling What to Expect pregnancy and parenting series that was written by the foundation's president, Heidi Murkoff, and her mother, the late Arlene Eisenberg.

This series of books has helped over 20 million families from pregnancies through their child's toddler years. "What to Expect When You're Expecting" is often referred to as America's pregnancy bible. According to a USA Today poll, it is read by 93 percent of all mothers that buy a pregnancy guide. The What to Expect series of books are not only the three best-selling parenting books in the country; they are among the best-selling books in the country on any topic. This week "What to Expect When You're Expecting" is number three on the New York Times Bestseller List.

But I am sorry to say, as many parents as the What to Expect books have helped, they have missed many more. As we know, our Nation's infant mortality rate is higher than 28 other countries. We are right behind Cuba. And even if a mother could afford to buy a prenatal guide she might not be able to read it. The literacy rate in the United States is a continuing problem. Today 21 to 23 percent or adults or some 40 to 44 million people across the country read at less than a fifth grade level.

Thus, the birth of the What to Expect Foundation, a new non-profit organization dedicated to helping mothers in need receive prenatal health and literacy education so they, too, can expect healthy pregnancies, safe deliveries, and can learn to become parents. We believe that a woman, when she becomes a mother, needs to learn how to read because a mother who can read can raise a child who can read.

The Basic Basics program provides prenatal education that takes into account the special health, economic, social and cultural needs of low-income women and gives prenatal providers culturally appropriate health literacy tools and support.

By 2003 we will have provided over 200,000 women across the country with the Baby Basics program in English and Spanish and we are now building Baby Basic model health literacy sites at prenatal clinics across the country.

While researching the Baby Basics book and program I had the opportunity to speak to hundreds of pregnant low-income women and the doctors, midwives, nurses, outreach workers, educators and social workers that care for them. From across the country I heard the pregnancy stories of the country's poorest women. Some of them were also the stories of just every woman—swollen feet, indigestion, back pain. Others were about hopes and fears that cut across income and education. Will I be a good mother? Will I know how to hold a child? Will I be able to provide for my baby?

But too many of these stories broke my heart. Teens who were pregnant because they wanted someone to love and to love them. Women pregnant with no health insurance, who worked long days for little income and hah to take off unpaid time to sit in a hard chair for hours waiting for an unscheduled five-minute free appointment at a crowded clinic. Women who saw a doctor for the first time the day their water broke because they could not afford care.

Secretary Thompson did an important thing and is to be congratulated when he realized that many pregnant women could not afford prenatal care. One look at the infant mortality rate and he did look for ways to fix it. He also realized that SCHIP, a dramatically successful program for families, had the funds and the ability to reach out to help in our constant battle against infant and maternal mortality. And I applaud him for finding a stopgap measure that was within his domain to help states provide prenatal care quickly and efficiently by extending the care to the fetus, with an implicit understanding that this was a quick fix, one that would be remedied by legislation.

Now, frankly, I am confused. In his recent letters to you, Senators, he seems to have changed his mind, saying such legislation is no longer needed; his quick fix is enough. But the quick fix put forward by the administration is not really a fix at all because now we have created even more problems. After we have spent so much time and money promoting prenatal care, we have gone and created an entirely new funded medical program called fetal care because fetal care and prenatal care are not the same thing. Please let me tell you why.

This September Secretary Thompson, Senator Kennedy and Senator Hatch, along with our foundation's president, Heidi Murkoff, spoke at Robert Wood Johnson's Covering Kids celebration honored SCHIP's fifth anniversary. Mothers and fathers explained how Child Health Plus helped their family. These were working families with two jobs working double shifts, to keep their families afloat.

One family, suddenly unemployed, had no idea how they were going to pay for their daughter's continuing diabetes care until they found out about SCHIP. Another hard-working mother spoke about SCHIP paying for surgery that saved her boy's life. These parents were heroes to their children and to the audience. With the help of SCHIP, they have provided for their families. Because SCHIP had been carefully crafted, marketed and promoted as help for working families and children, these parents were able to retain their dignity and were proud of their ability as parents to provide the health care their child needed when they needed it. Just as offering prenatal care to a woman can help her afford to do the best for her unborn child, it is friendly help that is offered with dignity and can be accepted with pride.

Offering fetal care? That is a slap in the face. This new regulation makes clear that fetal care is about the fetus first. Extras, like epidurals and pain medication, will only be available if a case can be made that they are for the health of the fetus. Fetal care offers the mother no dignity, devaluing her life, which she has risked by sharing her body with an unborn child.

Prenatal care acknowledges that there are two things that grow when a woman becomes pregnant. First, of course, there is the fetus, growing to become a healthy baby. And second, no less importantly, there is the woman, who must also grow. She must grow to think of herself as a mother, a parent, a provider. Inextricably linked in a dance as old as creation, mother and child grow together, both nurtured with love and care.

Fetal care unbinds those ties, breaks those bonds. It is about the government choosing fetuses over women, providing the fetus with all of its health care needs while saying to the woman we cannot help you.

Prenatal care provides a woman with the comprehensive health coverage she needs to have a baby. It cares for her body and her health. It helps her stay strong so she can be strong as a mother. It provides for her needs before and after the delivery and gives her the chance to recover so she has the strength and the health to nurse her precious new bundle.

Fetal care tells mothers that once they have had the baby, they are on their own. Like Cinderella after the ball, once the baby is delivered, no more fairy godmother. Suddenly her health care is gone. No glass slipper. Even her 48 hours guaranteed hospital stay is out of the picture.

Prenatal care is about family values. It helps create parents. It does what Early Head Start, Head Start, Healthy Start and Even Start do so well. It gives parents the strong shoulders they need to make sure no child is left behind. It fosters optimism.

Fetal care throws the parent out with the bathwater. It fosters pessimism and an early pervading sense of failure. From the start, it fails to acknowledge that a parent is a child's first and best teacher. To me, fetal care fosters foster care.

Prenatal care fills hospital wards with healthy babies. Fetal care fills hospitals with wards of the State.

Senators, so many good things can happen when a woman gets proper comprehensive prenatal care, as you have heard from my colleagues. The What to Expect Foundation links prenatal care to literacy training so women learn how to read and learn how to read to their babies. Healthy Start and other programs across the country are linking prenatal care to all kinds of positive self-esteem-building social programs—parenting skills, job training, long-term housing planning, financial planning.

We have trouble in this country getting women into prenatal care. Why would we ever want to put any barriers to prenatal care up?

Secretary Thompson has done an honorable thing by opening the door to prenatal care for thousands of women each year but imaginary barriers, liberal barriers, conservative barriers, unintended barriers, no matter what we want to call these barriers, regardless of their politics or their intent, they are unnecessary barriers to care.

I am here to tell you that hundreds of providers, practically every doctor, midwife and nurse across the country agrees that this fetal care quick-fix must not stand as a barrier. And every mother, including this mother, and the mothers who have told millions of mothers across the country what to expect, agree. Our job is to knock down the barriers. Passing S. 724 will remove those barriers. Then we can roll up our sleeves and get back to work because only a healthy parent can provide a healthy future for a healthy child. Thank you.

Senator BINGAMAN. Thank you very much.

Dr. Riley, you are the clean-up hitter on this panel. We are anxious to hear from you, too.

Dr. RILEY. These are hard acts to follow.

Thank you, Mr. Chairman, and members of the HELP Committee. As an obstetrician-gynecologist, I welcome the opportunity to speak with you this morning on behalf of the American College of Obstetricians and Gynecologists, 45,000 partners in women's health care. I look forward to discussing measures that will increase access to medical services for pregnant women.

I would first like to thank you, Senator Bingaman, for your leadership on this issue. I would also like to thank and acknowledge Senators Lincoln and Corzine for appearing before the committee today and for their commitment to uninsured women.

My name is Dr. Laura Riley and I am an assistant professor of obstetrics and gynecology at Harvard Medical School and the medical director of labor and delivery at Massachusetts General Hospital in Boston. I also chair the Committee on Obstetric Practice at ACOG.

I am pleased and honored to speak before the committee today on an issue that is extremely important to me. The focus of today's hearing is to discuss how being uninsured can impact maternal and fetal morbidity and mortality. For uninsured pregnant women, lack of prenatal and postpartum services can have devastating and lasting effects on both the mother and her fetus. There is no question that increasing access to prenatal care and appropriate postpartum services is of the utmost importance.

Unfortunately, one of great barriers to this care remains lack of insurance. I believe passage of Senate Bill 724, the Mothers and Newborns Health Insurance Act of 2001, would help us achieve this important goal. ACOG strongly supports S. 724, a bipartisan comprehensive bill that permits states to extend health coverage to pregnant women, enabling them to have full access to a range of services, including perinatal and postpartum medical care, and urge the Senate to quickly pass this legislation. ACOG, along with the Academy of Pediatrics, spells out recommendations for prenatal and postpartum care for the mother and the fetus in Guidelines for Perinatal Care, Fifth Edition. If we pass S. 724, we can deliver this care to many underserved and uninsured women.

I would like to take a moment to comment on the Department of Health and Human Services' recently issued regulation that allows states to provide prenatal and delivery benefits under the SCHIP program to mothers and the fetus, regardless of the mother's immigration status. We appreciate the administration's interest in expanding prenatal coverage to uninsured pregnant women. Their efforts to extend access is appreciated. However, this regulation, as it stands, raises some questions.

We at ACOG believe that it is unrealistic to exclude the mother and provide services solely to the fetus. It is impossible to separate mother-baby pairs and expect a good outcome for either of them. Our three principal concerns are the need for postpartum care, the need for essential components of prenatal care, and the logistical problems of implementing the administration's proposed legislation.

ACOG is very concerned that mothers will not have access to appropriate postpartum services. The rule clearly states that "Care after delivery, such as postpartum services, could not be covered because they are not services for an eligible child." Physicians regard postpartum care as essential for the health of the mother and the child.

Covering the fetus as opposed to the mother also raises questions of whether certain services will be available during pregnancy and labor if the condition is one that principally affects the woman. Postpartum care is especially critical for women who have preexisting medical complications and for those whose medical conditions were induced by their pregnancies, such as gestational diabetes or hypertension. Even women with uneventful deliveries and recoveries can develop conditions postpartum that require extra visits or even surgery. A woman may go home feeling well and return with problems.

I recently treated a 20-year-old Hispanic woman 8 days after an apparently uncomplicated vaginal delivery. She complained of 2 days of severe headache. Her blood pressure was 200 over 115 and upon arrival to the hospital, she suffered a grand mal seizure. There are many more stories like this, some even more tragic. Clearly when new mothers develop postpartum complications, quick access to medical care is absolutely critical.

I would also like to touch upon a population that may be most at risk for developing complications during and after pregnancy and why we must ensure that obstacles do not prevent them from seeking care. African-American women, Hispanic women who have immigrated to the United States, and American Indian and Alaskan native women are at greatest risk for maternal mortality.

The statistics are startling. CDC notes that African-American women are four times as likely to die of pregnancy complications compared with white women and American Indian and Alaskan native women are nearly twice as likely to die. In a 14-year national study of pregnancy-related deaths in the United States, CDC found that the pregnancy-related mortality ratio for African-American women was 25.1 deaths per 100,000 live births and 10.3 deaths per 100,000 live births for Hispanic women, versus six per 100,000 live births for white women. Poverty and lack of insurance clearly and certainly play a significant role in these alarming statistics. We are concerned that women without postpartum coverage, the very women that need the most help and who experience the highest rate of maternal morbidity and mortality, will be disproportionately affected.

As I have stated before, prenatal and intrapartum services are essential. It is inconceivable that there are diseases that affect the mother principally and have no overall effect on the fetus. Diseases such as diabetes and hypertension clearly have defined fetal effects. Maternal obesity, which requires nutrition counseling, behavioral interventions, and anesthesia consultation, is not a health condition limited to the mother.

For example, another patient of mine in her 8 month of pregnancy arrived in the emergency room clutching her head with pain and developed confusion over time. A CT scan revealed a large brain tumor. Yes, this is a maternal condition but you can imagine that the effects of neurosurgery and postoperative pain management all had an impact on her developing fetus.

Finally, Mr. Chairman, I want to share our concerns about the implementation of the administration's regulation and the impact it will have on OB-GYN practices. Already the health care system prevents physicians from spending needed time with patients. Skyrocketing medical liability premiums, onerous regulatory paperwork, and continued Medicare payment cuts can dramatically undermine our ability to serve our patients. All of these factors have combined to limit access to care and we urge Congress to support efforts to address these issues, as well.

I fear this regulation will create even more bureaucracy and red tape for physicians. For my patient who was 8 months pregnant with a brain tumor, figuring out which components of her care would be covered by such restrictive services would be an impossible task. Because this regulation also limits coverage to services directly related to the health of the fetus, OB-GYNs will be unsure whether medically necessary care can be covered. In most cases physicians will simply provide the care and deal with the coverage issues later, knowing that a tremendous amount of staff time and effort will be expended to recover minimal payment.

Furthermore, pregnant women may wonder if even they have the ability to access coverage for nonobstetric conditions or injuries and decide simply to not seek treatment. This uncertainty about coverage will discourage physicians from participating and deter women from seeking appropriate necessary care.

Mr. Chairman, in closing, I urge the Senate to quickly pass S. 724. I also encourage the administration to support enactment of this bill to expand coverage to uninsured pregnant women, ensuring access to comprehensive prenatal and postpartum coverage. It is the right thing to do. Thank you.

Senator BINGAMAN. Thank you very much.

[The prepared statement of Dr. Riley may be found in additional material.]

Senator BINGAMAN. I thank all four witnesses for just excellent testimony.

Before we start some questions let me defer to Senator Corzine for any comments or statements that he would like to make.

Senator CORZINE. Thank you, Mr. Chairman. Again let me congratulate you and compliment you on your leadership on this issue throughout this year and over a long period of time. Universal access to health care is certainly something that I think all of us would like to see but if we do not have the ability to provide that, providing it to the Nation's children and pregnant women is something that I think all of us can believe needs to be done.

I have a lengthy statement I will put into the record but I do want to reemphasize that we are creating controversy where there need be none. We are creating confusion, as we just heard Dr. Riley talk about, for our medical community where there need be none. And we are creating an unbelievable conflict between the health of the mother and the health of the fetus that need not be done. So I hope that we can resolve this and move forward quickly with respect to it.

I thank the witnesses for their testimony. It is far more articulate than I can be with regard to this, but this is something that I think the Nation ought to put high on its agenda and address quickly.

Senator BINGAMAN. So thank you very much to all of you and your excellent testimony.

Thank you very much, Senator Corzine, for your strong advocacy of this legislation here throughout this Congress.

Let me start with a couple of questions and then defer to Senator Lincoln and Senator Corzine for questions they have. First I wanted to allude to a very disturbing statistic that I am well aware of and that is that when you look at the various states in the Nation as to who has the biggest problem with regard to women of child-bearing age lacking appropriate insurance, my State of New Mexico is first in the Nation. There are 32 percent of the women of child-bearing age in New Mexico who do not have insurance coverage. Second to New Mexico is Texas. Twenty-eight percent of the women of child-bearing age there do not have any insurance coverage.

So it is a very serious problem and, of course, the statistics in our State I think add to or contribute to the very unfortunate national statistics that several witnesses have referred to.

Let me just ask any of you, starting with Dr. Green, I think the concern that I have had and a major motivation for introducing the legislation I introduced in this Congress and supporting Senator Bond's legislation, along with my colleagues, has been trying to deal with this problem of high mortality of newborns, high mortality of women in the delivery process. This legislation seemed to be the most effective thing we could do at the national level to try to deal with this.

Is there something else? Is there something other than passage of this type of legislation that would also be a significant contributor to solving this problem? I think we are sort of looking to you as experts to tell us what can be done to deal with these problems. I did not know if any of you have insights as to whether this is the most effective thing or whether there are others that we ought to be pursuing, as well.

Dr. Green, did you have any thoughts on that?

Dr. GREEN. Thank you. I think a number of the states have already identified that between Medicaid and SCHIP coverage, that is a lot of families affected who can be covered effectively by those programs. In fact, many states have increased the threshold for eligibility for SCHIP to 185 percent and in some states 200 percent of the poverty level.

So I guess the theme of my suggestion would be the increase in coverage both from Medicaid and through SCHIP and to that end then, this bill would be serving.

Senator BINGAMAN. Let me put a chart up that we have that tries to show the problem in my State. I asked Bruce Lesley, who has been the great champion on this, to put this chart together. The thatched part up at the right starting after age 18 is the area that we are trying to cover through this legislation. Medicaid does cover people up to 185 percent of poverty in my State. The SCHIP program covers anyone up to 235 percent of poverty through age 18 but then after that, of course, there is no coverage once a person is 19 years old, so we believe that this is an option that should be available to our State to pick up.

Dr. GREEN. The March of Dimes commissioned a study from Emory University to estimate the potential number of eligible pregnant women who could be covered by this legislation that gives states the option to enroll income-eligible pregnant women in the SCHIP program. Those estimates are 41,000 women nationwide would be eligible for coverage under this bill.

The Congressional Budget Office has recently released some estimates of their own—about 30,000 newly eligible pregnant women could be covered. So between 30,000 and 40,000 women could be affected by this regulation. That is a lot of families.

Senator BINGAMAN. Right. Very good.

Let me ask Dr. Riley, you went into some depth about the problems that you see with trying to sort out what is covered under this new regulation that has been issued and Senator Corzine just referred to that sort of needless complication that we are adding to the system for physicians and all.

Two, I think that you mentioned are diabetes and hypertension, questions about whether those kinds of things would be covered. Would you want to elaborate on that at all as to how you think obstetricians would make those decisions?

Dr. RILEY. I think that obstetricians are going to have a tough time deciding what component of treatment for hypertension is going to get covered because it directly relates to the fetus, yet this part is really for the mom's long-term health.

Hypertension may not even be the best example. I think a very good example is my patient with the brain tumor. I mean the brain tumor was not going to affect her fetus directly but certainly the neurosurgery that we did and lowering her core body temperature probably had some effect on her fetus.

I think that there are definitely going to be some medical illnesses that complicate pregnancies for which you cannot separate the mother and the baby. You may not be able to define the fetal effect but there is probably a fetal effect. I do not think that we want to allow physicians to then be more confused and start making arbitrary decisions about what treatment they will give and what treatment they will not give.

Senator BINGAMAN. Dr. Bucciarelli, did you have any thoughts on this? You are in the business of providing pediatric care.

Dr. BUCCIARELLI. Right. I agree with agree Dr. Riley. When we go into a delivery room or we go in consultation with the perinatologist, we are working on a unique situation in which there are two lives that are inexorably bound together and there is virtually nothing that I can think of that would affect the mother and not directly or indirectly affect the fetus.

One of the examples given earlier is if a mother breaks an arm, how does that affect the fetus? Well, the stress, the hormones that are put out when somebody has that kind of injury cross the placenta and those kinds of hormones, small peptides, greatly affect blood flow and very commonly blood flow to the brain, which is what we are trying to preserve. We have babies that are born with a completely normal delivery process that have devastating defects in the long run, probably because of these kinds of things, stresses in the mom that we are not aware of.

So I just cannot think of anything that would go on in a mom that would not directly or indirectly affect the fetus and I would agree with Dr. Riley that separating those two would make it so difficult to take care of these patients.

Senator BINGAMAN. Senator Lincoln, go ahead with any questions you have.

Senator LINCOLN. Thank you, Mr. Chairman.

Well, a little bit to expand on that, when you talk about that you cannot think of anything that would be different or where you could separate those two, my understanding of the regulation is that it would be left up to the states. So basically you are going to have different states deciding what is covered, what is not, different care given to mothers depending on where they live and where they seek services and all of a sudden you are going to have physicians again trying to make these decisions. Is this a procedure that I follow the clinical guidelines, which you all obviously have clinical guidelines, or do I follow another path or another pattern because I want to take care of both of these but I cannot do it and get reimbursed or get paid for services in that way.

To me, that sounds enormously confusing and I cannot imagine that physicians, particularly in light of some of what Dr. Riley has brought up in regard to liability that we have seen with obstetrics and gynecology and other difficulties that they have, I mean what do you all see in terms of the confusion, the logistical complications that this would present and finally, I guess, perhaps the lack of reimbursement or the knowledge of that for whether it is prenatal or postpartum care? How his that going to affect the willingness of providers to actually serve or participate in these SCHIP programs?

Dr. RILEY. I think that it will lead to more and more physicians not participating at all. It is too much paperwork. It is too much confusion. You leave yourself open to a great deal of liability, giving half the care you should give. I think that people will just say I do not want to take care of this segment of the population.

Then again it will get us right back to where we started from, where there is lack of access.

Senator LINCOLN. It is so counterproductive to what we want to accomplish.

Dr. RILEY. Absolutely.

Senator LINCOLN. Dr. Bucciarelli, I know I delivered at a university hospital and I can remember my father, who is a wonderful man but he is a basic dirt farmer from East Arkansas. I had never seen my father cry until I went up to the neonatal intensive care unit with him, took him up to see one of our twins, who had to spend about 24 hours under some oxygen from a pneumothorax, and we were very fortunate. I went full term. The boys were big, good size babies and all of that, but right next to Bennett was a twin. They were born at, I think, like 24 weeks, 25 weeks, maybe even 23 weeks, and one of the twins survived; one of them did not.

It was incredible to see that baby and as I said, I had never seen my father cry until he looked at that child. The comment that he said, which was not only is that amazing to see, but he said that poor individual is going to have complications all his life.

When we talk about the lack of prenatal care and we talk about how important it is for the health of the family and the child we are not just talking about delivery. We are not just talking about postpartum. Can you kind of expand on some of the things, too, when you have a delivery without the adequate prenatal care and without the adequate postpartum care, what do we see in developing pediatrics and in children down the line in terms of developmental disabilities and other health care complications, even the statistics on incarceration, when you are talking about those kinds of situations?

Dr. BUCCIARELLI. Well, there can be a life-time loss for the family and the child. Certainly the age group that you refer to have a high mortality and those that survive often have some disabilities, from mild to very severe. But, you know, although I marvel when I am in the NICU, as well, at the advances that we have made but I am absolutely convinced that we get handed a healthier baby and it makes my job easier because of what is happening in obstetrics and gynecology and the prenatal care, the intrapartum care gives me a child that is healthier and allows me to use the technology that is available.

So 10 years ago we had a lot of the technology we have today but that child would not survive. The difference is the prenatal care, the ability to treat these kinds of conditions of high blood pressure and disability, so the obstetrician hands me a baby that is screaming, pink, and almost ready to feed.

May I just make one other comment that I think you alluded to? That is the issue of breast feeding. That is so important in the outcome of children, that they get the right kind of initial exposure to immunoglobulins to decrease the amount of infections, to allow their gut to develop appropriately. And we have made great strides in our country in having women breast feed and that is purely a postpartum service. You do not talk about breast feeding in prenatal care, maybe a little during the delivery, but it is a postpartum service and without coverage for lactation consultants and without coverage of the physician's time to talk to the mother about breast feeding, breast feeding in our country will disappear very, very rapidly and it will be a tremendous loss to the health of our children.

Senator LINCOLN. That is so true. I can remember asking to be able to see a lactation consultant and they said, "What?" It is interesting.

Miss Bernstein, thank you so much for such a moving statement. I have to say that I was one of those millions of women who had "What to Expect When You're Expecting" on my shelf. I have read it and I was very interested to see my husband, who happens to be an OB-GYN, how much he enjoyed reading it. We did read it together. It was something that provided us, I think, a great perspective on many of the different things we would see. He certainly knew the medical aspects but for me it was a tremendous help when I was carrying my sons. But, as you've said, not all women have been so lucky to be able to read the book or get the kind of prenatal care that they need.

In my home State of Arkansas there are about 97,000 women of child-bearing age, between 15 and 24, who do not have health insurance. We rank 35th in the Nation in this regard and when you look at Senator Bingaman's chart there, we only cover 133 percent of poverty in Medicaid and we go to 200 percent of poverty with SCHIP.

But you talked a bit about the effects that providing health care to only the fetus would have on mothers. I would like for you maybe to share with us from your experience with Baby Basics programs and the people that you have met, maybe describe some hypothetical situations concerning pregnant women. Or maybe you have some situations that you have in mind that you have seen that you would like to share, some low-income, maybe some that do not speak English, perhaps.

Ms. BERNSTEIN. I think this brings kind of an answer to Senator Bingaman, also, that I would like to talk about. One of the things that I have noticed about access to care, to early childhood care and prenatal care, is that a lot of people do not know what does exist for them. A lot of mothers come in late because they do not know their rights. They do not know what is available.

One of the things that I have watched with SCHIP that is a marvelous program is that families do not know it is for them. They do not know that they can get this and it is not until by accident they hear—I mean I have heard stories of people hearing about it on the radio by accident and realizing, oh, wait, I fit into that.

One of the things I think we should think about is when this is successful, which I hope it will be, how we can use this as a continuum of care because women do go in for prenatal care and you do not sign them up for SCHIP; they do not find out about it. With this, we have expanded the entry to the SCHIP program. You get pregnant women in there and you get them signed up with their children and then you have expanded the SCHIP program to reach the thousands of families that we have been unable to reach.

I think that what I have learned from doing this Baby Basics program, and I will tell a story that Heidi Murkoff and I watched happen together. We are at Reikers Island at a parenting program and this was really the impetus for starting the program. We gave out copies of "What to Expect When You're Expecting" to pregnant mothers in prison, who dove into these books. They looked like every middle class mother I have ever seen who immediately wants to know everything that is going on inside their bodies because an alien life is growing. It is a shocking and exciting and a marvelous time and you want to know everything.

A woman at the end walked up. She was emaciated except for a swollen belly and it was pretty clear that she probably had been just incarcerated and was there for drug use and was probably getting the best care she had ever had because she was in prison. She asked Heidi, "They told me I need to have an x-ray of my tooth and I just read in the book that it's going to hurt the baby. Should I have one?"

And we could not help but stop and say this woman probably was not eating, she was probably doing crack cocaine. This was a few years ago. She loved her baby. She had no idea—she came from a different world than I came from. She did not know what to do to help her baby. She did not know what it was going to take to have a healthy pregnancy. Once we started giving her the information, once we started showing her what she needed to do, she was as eager as any mother.

Much of it is about access, about education. The things that we think come naturally that you know, whether it is nutrition, whether it is basic hygiene, if you did not grow up with that, you do not even know to begin there. To deny that to a mother is an awful thing to do to the mother because she wants to make that baby healthy. The more help and the more information you can give her, the more that she will take control. She will become a parent, which is really what our goal is.

That, I guess, is the point of what I am saying, is the more that you take that control away from the mother, the less that she will grow to take that responsibility. And I think that is what our goal should be, is to create parents, not just healthy babies, but to create parents who can give their babies that health.

Senator LINCOLN. That is a continuing thing.

Thank you, Mr. Chairman. I may have another one but I would like to give my colleague over there an opportunity.

Senator BINGAMAN. All right, Senator Corzine?

Senator CORZINE. Thank you, Mr. Chairman.

I do not really feel like asking the question I am going to ask after that statement because I think that is really getting at the heart of the matter of how we bring our kids into the system and how we frame their futures and their lives, but let me ask a bureaucratic question. Dr. Bucciarelli or Dr. Green may be the appropriate source.

The administration argues that states can apply for waivers in this process. New Jersey is a State that has done this. Checking with the people who are responsible, it was difficult. Dr. Bucciarelli, Florida's Healthy Kids program, I guess, has done the same. Do you think this will be a procedure that will flow smoothly and easily under the regulations and therefore this legislation is unneeded or what will be the difficulties, the stops, the road blocks? Aside from the other issues about confusions that come into doctors' minds, what will be the confusions in the states and the conflicts? Any of the panelists can comment on that.

Dr. BUCCIARELLI. Well, in regard to the waivers, we have had experience in filing other waivers in the State of Florida. They were very complicated. They took a long time before we got through. It was, I think, a significant waste of money and time in administration in doing that. When something like this can be done by legislation as an option, purely as an option, without having to go through all that process, to me, it makes more sense to allow the states to take an option to be able to move that, instead of going through the waiver process.

Dr. GREEN. I would like to add an additional comment to that important statement just made. That is that with the legislation, then Federal funding becomes available to the states and, as we all know, states are not exactly flush these days. So I think when we talk about something as critical as health care coverage for our vulnerable citizens, then the additional financial incentive from the Federal support of the program through the legislation would be enormously important.

Senator CORZINE. I suspect we all understand the difference between authorization and appropriation and it is even more difficult when you are applying for waivers where there is lacking an authorization.

One other slight difference. Aside from the judgmental issues that I think really get at the heart of a controversy that need not be, do I understand it correctly that the administration's program only attends to the newborn child for 3 months, as opposed to a year, which is the element that is involved in the legislation? What are we missing as we look after our children in the start of their life along these lines? Anyone on the panel.

Dr. BUCCIARELLI. Certainly there is a tremendous amount of information that says the first year of life is critical to the child's health and further development and the American Academy of Pediatrics for some time has been a proponent of presumptive eligibility and continuous eligibility through that first year of life to allow immunizations to be done on time and the other kinds of well visits for not only screening but diagnosis and treatment of conditions. Certainly within the first 3 months a lot of that will be known but after that it certainly will not. And as I understand the legislation, it is a year coverage but it could go back to early pregnancy or conception, so 9 months of the year is covered at that time and then there are only 3 months afterwards.

I think a good example, if I might, is the issue with hearing impairment. Most states have a requirement to do hearing screening and they are done in the newborn period. But to be able to diagnosis carefully and treat a hearing disability, you have to do that several months later. It is critical that that be done before 6 months of age because if it is not done before 6 months of age, there are long-term losses with reading, language, that may never be recovered.

So if you screen the baby in the newborn period and it is covered but it is not covered after 3 months and they are on and off or they fall off for a variety of administrative reasons and never come back, you have wasted time and effort in screening that child. Plus, without the proper diagnosis and treatment, we have lost an opportunity to allow a child to develop to their fullest potential, and that is a serious loss.

Senator CORZINE. Anyone else want to comment?

Dr. RILEY. I would just add yet another example that comes to my mind because it is my area of research but the diagnosis of HIV infection in a newborn is a difficult one to make. You might start to make the diagnosis at birth but then really you have to repeat the studies at 4 months of age to be absolutely sure that you have made the correct diagnosis. Certainly these are children, just a small segment of the population, but these are children that the care in the first year of life really will determine how well they do and it is not a case of how well they do but whether they live or die and I think that it would be horrible to go backwards on all the strides we have made in medicine for this group of children.

Senator CORZINE. Let me ask sort of a medical question. Is it typical that children have all their immunizations applied in the first 3 months?

Dr. BUCCIARELLI. No. In fact, at that point we are just beginning to get into the immunizations that would go on. Most of the primary immunizations are done at the end of the first year but even after that there are other immunizations that are important. So that continuous coverage, continuous eligibility, is critical to make sure children do get the series of immunizations they need and that they get them on time.

Senator CORZINE. Thank you, Mr. Chairman. I think we see some of the reasons why this is so important.

Senator BINGAMAN. Well, thank you very much.

Let me just ask another question or two here and then if either Senator Lincoln or Senator Corzine have more, we will obviously hear those.

I wanted to put up a chart that is very hard for anyone to read from the back of the room. If you can read that, we certainly will give you some kind of award. I have given each of the witnesses a copy of this. What we have tried to do here is to set out aspects of the regulation, first of all, and then of the legislation, as well, in several areas where we think the legislation provides coverage and provides benefits that the regulation does not. I wanted to just mention what those are.

Obviously coverage of prenatal care and labor and delivery, that is clearly covered under our legislation. The coverage is mixed, as we have discussed here, under the regulation. Coverage of postpartum care is clearly covered under the legislation, not covered under the regulation by its own language. Prohibition on waiting periods for pregnant women, that again we have made provision in the legislation to ensure that there are no waiting periods involved. Obviously if you are pregnant you need care; you do not need to wait 6 months or a year.

Prohibition on cost-sharing for pregnant women. Again we have made it clear in the legislation that states would not be permitted to require any cost-sharing. And then this issue about whether or not the child would be eligible for coverage or covered for the first 12 months of life and we think that is an important benefit of the legislation.

Finally, the one Dr. Green has mentioned here and Dr. Bucciarelli I think maybe, as well, that our legislation does provide funds. We have identified ways to fund this additional coverage, which I think should be a substantial benefit to states because no such funding is provided in the regulation.

Let me just ask again on this waiver issue, it strikes me as sort of perverse that we are saying to states, which I think is the administration's position—I had a conversation frankly with Deputy Assistant Secretary Claude Allen on the phone where his position was if states want to provide this coverage to pregnant women, it is not a problem; they can just seek a waiver.

It strikes me first of all that it is a little perverse to have a legal structure where if you want to provide coverage to pregnant women you have to get a waiver; the provisions of law that normally apply need to be waived. This is not an experimental kind of a program, as I understand it. I mean we are pretty clear that these benefits are real; they have been real for a long time.

The regulation says the secretary's ability to intervene through one mechanism—that is, a waiver—should not be the sole option for states and may, in fact, be an inferior option, which I think is certainly a clear statement, a correct statement. Then it says waivers are discretionary on the part of the secretary and time-limited while State plan amendments are permanent and subject to allotment neutrality.

I would also just point out for the record here that the National Governors Association is on record. They have issued a policy that states, "The governors call on Congress to create a State option that would allow states to provide health coverage to income-eligible women under SCHIP. This small shift in Federal policy would allow states to provide critical prenatal care, would increase the likelihood that children born to SCHIP mothers would have a healthy start."

So I do not know if any of you have other comments on this notion that the waiver is a good option. It does not strike me as a very good option for states to go in and say please waive the applicable laws and let us cover pregnant women.

Have any of you focussed on that to any greater extent than this? No one seems to—Ms. Bernstein, did you have any comment?

Ms. BERNSTEIN. I was going to say that I think if you did a survey of middle class mothers across the country, they all think that prenatal care is paid for for everyone. I think that most people in this country who do not live in fear of getting health coverage have no idea that we turn people away every day. The thought of a waiver is that same way of thinking. This is a right. Prenatal care should be something that is provided for in this country and to have to get a waiver to be allowed to do it is bad wording. It is embarrassing, I think.

Senator BINGAMAN. Well, I thought the wording in your testimony to the effect that fetal care involves throwing the parent out with the bath water, I thought that was a good way to put it.

Ms. BERNSTEIN. Thank you.

Senator BINGAMAN. Let me call on Senator Lincoln for any additional questions she has.

Senator LINCOLN. Thank you, Mr. Chairman.

Dr. Green, following on that question, I think it is interesting. I kind of wanted to find out where the March of Dimes was and how active they are at the State level or are there any plans to be active to encourage states to expand coverage to pregnant women in what we have talked about here? I mean we know that the waiver—I agree with the chairman that the waiver process and what we are talking about there is pretty counterproductive to what we really want to be doing but it is an option that if you are faced with, whether you use the regulation that the administration is giving us or you go for the waiver, which is the most productive to encourage states to go toward?

Dr. GREEN. Well, the March of Dimes has a chapter, at least one chapter in every State, in Puerto Rico and in the District of Columbia and I think that you are aware, Senator Lincoln, of the energy emanating from these chapters at the State level with respect to advocacy.

Senator LINCOLN. Absolutely.

Dr. GREEN. So I think that the March of Dimes is active in this program on two levels. One is certainly if states did not have the option to expand SCHIP to encompass pregnant women, then our chapters would be very active in trying to help those State legislatures to apply for this waiver program.

Senator LINCOLN. If they do not have S. 724.

Dr. GREEN. If they did not have S. 724, exactly. As you have heard, it would be enormously expensive in terms of resources, time, energy. In fact, we would prefer to have passage of S. 724 so that we can focus our attention on another level of this kind of issue, namely getting parents, getting women, getting children enrolled in the programs that already exist because, as we have heard in the news, many states do not have complete implementation of their SCHIP program because families do not know about it, there are lots of barriers, language, literacy, logistics.

So our chapters are prepared to help states apply for waivers but we would really rather help the communities get the coverage that they deserve. We will do both if we have to.

Senator LINCOLN. Right. But what I am hearing you say is that if you have the choice—if the legislation that we are talking about today is not made into law and states are not given that option to make that choice, then the March of Dimes would not encourage states to take up the option of covering an unborn child. They are going to encourage states to take the more difficult option because it is more comprehensive, because you know that the outcome for the child, for the mother, for the family, for the community and the Nation are all going the be better if we get more comprehensive care.

Dr. GREEN. That is absolutely right, that access to coverage for children and pregnant women is one of our major foundation priorities, so we will certainly work with states to apply for those waivers and we applaud Colorado for their slogging through the process.

Senator LINCOLN. Just one comment, Mr. Chairman, and I will be finished. There has been a lot of talk about the availability and the knowledge, the education of people about what is available. We did try a couple of years ago with some legislation which we did pass to try and make the SCHIP program a little bit more available in the sense that we could publicize it and get better ways of getting the message out there, whether it is one-stop shopping or making sure that we have brochures and information out there in the appropriate places, like pediatricians' offices or in other places, as well, in our DHS offices and other things.

So we have tried to do some of that but if you have other suggestions, please let us know because we do not need to stop there. We know we have not completed what we need to do, but we have made an initial step. So I would encourage you to continue that dialogue with us.

Thank you, Mr. Chairman.

Senator BINGAMAN. Well, thank you and again thank all of the witnesses. I think it has been very useful testimony and we will obviously have an opportunity when Congress comes back into session once again to pass this legislation. I know Senator Lincoln and I and Senator Corzine and Senator Bond will be making that effort again and we hope that we can succeed with the legislation before Congress adjourns.

Thank you very much and that will conclude the hearing.

[Additional material follows:]

ADDITIONAL MATERIAL

PREPARED STATEMENT OF NANCY GREEN, M.D.

Mr. Chairman, I am Nancy Green and I am the Medical Director for the March of Dimes Birth Defects Foundation. I am pleased to be here today to discuss with you the importance of providing all pregnant women access to health insurance coverage and a comprehensive set of maternity services. I want to salute you, Mr. Chairman, and seventeen of your colleagues for sponsoring legislation that would give states the option of covering income eligible pregnant women 19 and older through State Children's Health Insurance Programs (SCHIP). We would like to especially thank Senators Bond, Lincoln and Corzine who recently joined you on the Senate floor to discuss the need for S. 724.

President Franklin Roosevelt established the March of Dimes in 1938 to fight polio. The March of Dimes committed funds for research and within 20 years Foundation grantees were successful in developing a vaccine to prevent polio. The March of Dimes then turned its attention to improving the health of children through the prevention of birth defects and infant mortality. As you might expect, providing coverage to both pregnant women and infants is a policy priority and especially pertinent to the advancement of our mission because in January we will launch a $75 million multi-year campaign to address the growing problem of prematurity.

Today, the Foundation has more than 3 million volunteers and 1,600 staff members who work through chapters in every state, the District of Columbia and Puerto Rico. We are a unique partnership of scientists, clinicians, parents, business leaders and other volunteers and we work to accomplish our mission by conducting and funding programs of research, community services, education and advocacy.

At the March of Dimes, our overarching goal is to improve the health of mothers and children. This is why we are so concerned about improving access to health coverage for pregnant women and their newborns.

THE PROBLEM OF THE UNINSURED

Mr. Chairman, lack of health coverage continues to be a significant problem for many Americans. The Census Bureau recently reported that 41 million Americans were uninsured in 2001. Particularly troubling, Census Bureau data commissioned by the March of Dimes show that in 2001, 11.5 million women (18.7 percent) or nearly one in five women of childbearing age (15-44) went without health insurance a higher rate than other Americans under age 65 (15.8 percent). That is, some 28 percent of uninsured Americans are women of childbearing age. Hispanic women in this age group are almost three times as likely as whites to be uninsured 38 percent compared to 13 percent respectively. Native American (30 percent), African-American (23 percent) and Asian (20 percent) women were also likelier than whites to be uninsured. New Mexico (32 percent) and Texas (28 percent) had the highest rates of uninsured women of childbearing age for the 1999-2001 period according to the U.S. Census Bureau, compared with a U.S average of 18 percent for these years.

Since the mid-1980's expanded Medicaid eligibility for pregnant women has resulted in better rates of coverage for them than for women in general. The Congressional Budget Office, citing in part March of Dimes supported research, estimates that about 1.7 million pregnancies are covered each year by Medicaid. But as the data indicate, considerable room for improvement remains.

HEALTH INSURANCE MAKES A DIFFERENCE

Numerous studies have shown that having insurance coverage affects how people use health care services. In particular, the uninsured are less likely to have a usual source of medical care and are more likely to delay or forgo needed health care services.

In a report issued earlier this year by the Institute of Medicine, researchers concluded that "[L]ike Americans in general, pregnant women's use of health services varies by insurance status. Uninsured women receive fewer prenatal care services than their insured counterparts and report greater difficulty in obtaining the care that they believe they need. Studies find large differences in use between privately insured and uninsured women and smaller differences between uninsured and publicly insured women." A study funded by the March of Dimes and cited by the Institute of Medicine in its report shows that some 18.1 percent of uninsured pregnant women in 1996 reported going without needed medical care during the year in which they gave birth. That compares with 7.6 percent of privately insured pregnant women and 8.1 percent of pregnant women covered by Medicaid.

Mr. Chairman, we know pregnancy represents a significant cost to young parents. These families, many of whom work in small businesses that don't provide health insurance, face significant costs even with the healthiest pregnancies, and for families with a problem pregnancy, the financial impact can be devastating. Without access to health insurance, many pregnant women will delay seeing a doctor and getting the prenatal care they need. As the report that accompanied legislation passed by the Senate Committee on Finance stated, "[R]ecent studies have shown that infants born to mothers receiving late or no prenatal care are more likely to face complications which can result in hospitalization, expensive medical treatments, and increased costs to public programs. Closing the gap in coverage between mothers and their children will improve the health of both, while reducing costs for taxpayers."

The March of Dimes' objective is to reduce the number of uninsured pregnant women and children and to improve access to medical care. As you know, the March of Dimes supports elimination of any income eligibility disparities between mothers and newborns. To meet this objective, the Foundation has worked throughout this Congress to obtain support for a modest, incremental step to help improve access to health services for uninsured pregnant women by amending SCHIP. We support giving states the flexibility they need to cover income-eligible pregnant women age 19 and older, and to automatically enroll infants born to SCHIP-eligible mothers. By establishing a uniform eligibility threshold for coverage for pregnant women and infants, states will be able to improve maternal health, eliminate waiting periods for infants and streamline administration of publicly supported health programs. Currently, according to the Department of Health and Human Services' Centers for Medicare and Medicaid Services and the National Governors' Association, 36 states and the District of Columbia have income eligibility thresholds that are more restrictive for women than for their newborns. Encouraging states to eliminate this disparity by allowing them to establish a uniform eligibility threshold for pregnant women and their infants should be a national policy priority.

Mr. Chairman, in January and on several occasions throughout the year, we were pleased that on behalf of the administration HHS Secretary Thompson endorsed legislation to achieve this important objective. However, the March of Dimes is disappointed to learn that the administration has apparently withdrawn its support for legislation and instead will rely on a regulation issued on October 2, 2002 that permits states to cover unborn children. Specifically, we are deeply concerned that final regulation fails to provide to the mother the standard scope of maternity care services recommended by the American College of Obstetricians and Gynecologists (ACOG) and the American Academy of Pediatrics (AAP). Of particular concern, the regulation explicitly states that postpartum care is not covered and, therefore, federal reimbursement will not be available for these services. In addition, because of the contentious collateral issues raised by this regulation groups like the March of Dimes will find it even more difficult to work in the states to generate support for legislation to extend coverage to uninsured pregnant women. We agree with the Secretary about the value of prenatal care to achieve healthy birth outcomes. In fact, as recently as January 31, 2002, Secretary Thompson has said that "[P]renatal care for women and their babies is a crucial part of the medical care every person should have throughout the life cycle. Prenatal services can be a vital, life-long determinant of health, and we should do everything we can to make this care available for all pregnant women. It is one of the most important investments we can make for the long-term good health of our nation." We couldn't agree more. When a new mother goes home following delivery, the March of Dimes wants to be sure that she is healthy enough to support herself, to breast feed and care for her newborn, and to participate fully in her family's life.

SOLUTIONS

Mr. Chairman, you and your Finance Committee colleagues approved S. 724, the "Mothers and Newborns Health Insurance Act of 2002," in early July and similar legislation is pending in the House of Representatives. By including important provisions from your bill, S. 1016, the "Start Healthy, Stay Healthy Act," the Finance Committee-approved legislation would accomplish these important policy priorities. By doing so it would bring the SCHIP program into alignment with every other federal health insurance program all of which extend coverage to pregnant women and their babies.

The provisions of S. 724 that are particularly important to advancing the mission of the March of Dimes are:

1. *Allowing states the flexibility to extend SCHIP coverage to pregnant women 19 and older.*

States would be able to receive federal financing to help provide health coverage for income-eligible pregnant women. No waiting period would apply for participation in the program, and coverage of the mother would extend for at least two months following the birth of the child the postpartum coverage timeframe recommended by the American College of Obstetricians and Gynecologists (ACOG) and the American Academy of Pediatrics (AAP). Estimates of the annual impact of this change in law suggest that some 30,000 to 40,000 uninsured pregnancies could be covered.

2. *Automatically enrolling newborns whose mothers are enrolled in SCHIP and 12 month continuous coverage*

Automatic enrollment of newborns is important to avoid gaps in coverage for medically vulnerable infants. Enrollment of infants born to mothers eligible for SCHIP should begin the moment the child is born. This is especially important when a baby is premature, has a birth defect, or is in other ways medically fragile. In addition to automatic enrollment in SCHIP, newborns would remain enrolled in the program for one year. Many of these newborns would be eligible for coverage under current law, but often are not enrolled on timely basis. S. 724 establishes continuity of care for infants by guaranteeing coverage for the first year of life when access to health care services is particularly important for a healthy start in life.

3. *Outreach Improvements*

In addition to the positive effects of enrolling pregnant women in SCHIP, S. 724 includes provisions to improve outreach. Research and state experience suggests that covering pregnant women is a highly successful outreach mechanism for enrolling older eligible children. Several states have found that expanding coverage to uninsured parents results in increased enrollment of eligible children (including California, Illinois, Kentucky, Nevada, Rhode Island, and Wisconsin).

CONCLUSION

At the March of Dimes we believe that improving access to health care for uninsured pregnant women and their infants should be a national priority. S. 724 has broad bipartisan support in both Houses of Congress and the National Governors' Association has called on Congress to give states this option. In addition, twenty-six national organizations have endorsed this initiative. In short, Mr. Chairman, S. 724 would give us, and other organizations committed to improving the health of women and children, the opportunity to work in states across the country to expand access to comprehensive maternity services as recommended by obstetricians and pediatric practitioners.

Once again, on behalf of the March of Dimes thank you for your commitment to improving the health of children and their families and for this opportunity to testify on the issues of critical importance to pregnant women and infants.

I would be pleased to answer any questions the Committee may have.

PREPARED STATEMENT OF LAURA E. RILEY, M.D.

Thank you, Mr. Chairman, and members of the Senate Health, Education, Labor and Pensions Committee, for holding this important hearing. As an obstetrician-gynecologist, I welcome the opportunity to speak with you this morning on behalf of the American College of Obstetricians and Gynecologist's (ACOG) 45,000 partners in women's health care. I look forward to discussing measures that will increase access to medical services for pregnant women.

I would like to also specifically thank Senators Bond, Bingaman, Lincoln and Corzine, and others, for their strong leadership on the issue of uninsured pregnant women. Your efforts to enact meaningful legislation are deeply appreciated.

My name is Dr. Laura Riley, and I am Assistant Professor of Ob/Gyn at Harvard Medical School and the Medical Director of Labor and Delivery at Massachusetts General Hospital in Boston. I also chair the Committee on Obstetric Practice at ACOG. I am pleased and honored to speak before the Committee today on an issue that is near and dear to me.

The focus of today's hearing is to discuss how being uninsured can impact maternal and infant mortality. For uninsured pregnant women, going without needed prenatal and postpartum services can have devastating and lasting effects on both the mother and fetus. I have seen firsthand the consequences of women whose first visit to a physician is in the emergency room upon delivery. I have also seen the effects of severe postpartum complications on the health of the mother, conditions which, unfortunately, disproportionately affect minority women. Many of these conditions could have been reduced or prevented had a physician seen them early in their pregnancy. By assuring insurance coverage, and increasing access to prenatal care and appropriate postpartum services, we can reduce complications. I believe passage of Senate Bill 724, the "Mothers and Newborns Health Insurance Act of 2001," would help us achieve this goal.

ACOG strongly supports S. 724, a bipartisan, comprehensive bill that extends coverage to pregnant women, introduced last year by Senators Christopher "Kit" Bond (R-MO) and John Breaux (D-LA) and supported by a number of Senators, including Jeff Bingaman (D-NM) and Blanche Lincoln (D-AR). S. 724 permits states to expand health coverage to pregnant women, enabling them to have full access to a range of services, including comprehensive prenatal and postpartum medical services, that promote healthy pregnancies and deliveries and healthy babies. We urge the Senate to quickly pass this legislation.

ACOG has long recognized that a full spectrum of health services is necessary to ensure uneventful pregnancies, healthy deliveries, and a postpartum period free of complications. Recommendations for care are spelled out in Guidelines for Perinatal Care, Fifth Edition, which was developed jointly by ACOG and the American Academy of Pediatrics. Guidelines provides a description of the components of prenatal and postpartum care that are important to both the fetus and the pregnant woman. If we can pass S. 724, we can deliver this care to many underserved and uninsured women and reduce instances of morbidity and mortality.

NEW SCHIP REGULATION

Recently, the Department of Health and Human Services (HHS) issued a regulation that allows states to provide prenatal care and delivery benefits under the State Children's Health Insurance Program (SCHIP) to mothers and fetuses regardless of the mother's immigration status. We appreciate the Administration's interest in expanding prenatal coverage to uninsured pregnant women. Increased access to prenatal services is essential in our fight to reduce maternal and infant mortality. There is no question that as a nation we must do better to address this incidence.

The Administration recognizes that prenatal care is essential to ensure healthy pregnancies, however the regulation's approach to achieve this goal is a cause for concern. In particular, ACOG has several principle concerns with the rule. We hope to work with both Congress and the Administration to address these issues.

POSTPARTUM CARE CRITICAL

ACOG is very concerned that mothers will not have access to postpartum services under the regulation. The rule clearly states that "care after delivery, such as postpartum services could not be covered as part of the Title XXI State Plan because they are not services for an eligible child."

The regulation also revises the definition of "child" under SCHIP to clarify that "an unborn child including the period from conception to birth may be considered a 'targeted low-income child.'" Limiting coverage to the fetus instead of the mother omits a critical component of postpartum care that physicians regard as essential for the health of the mother and child. Covering the fetus as opposed to the mother also raises questions of whether certain services will be available during pregnancy and labor if the condition is one that more directly affects the woman.

The best way to address this coverage issue is to pass S. 724, supported by Senators Bond, Bingaman and Lincoln and many others, and which provides a full range of medical services during and after pregnancy directly to the pregnant woman. Early access to prenatal care can help determine if a mother is at risk, but comprehensive follow-up care is also vital to avoid further complications. Pregnancy can sometimes signal the onset of new conditions such as diabetes or hypertension that require careful attention to the mother and child. When new mothers develop postpartum complications, quick access to their physicians is absolutely critical.

Postpartum care is especially important for women who have preexisting medical conditions, and for those whose medical conditions were induced by their pregnancies, such as gestational diabetes or hypertension, and for whom it is necessary to ensure that their conditions are stabilized and treated. A wide range of diseases may affect the mother during and after pregnancy, such as cardiac disease, pulmonary embolism and renal disease; postpartum monitoring is critical is these cases.

Women can go home well and return with problems. I recently treated a 20-year-old Hispanic woman eight days after an apparently uncomplicated delivery. She complained of two days of headache; she had a blood pressure of 200/115 and, upon arrival at the hospital suffered a seizure. Another 28-year-old woman had an emergent cesarean delivery. She went home and returned later with fever and abdominal pain. She remained in the hospital for 13 days on intravenous antibiotics to treat bacteria in her blood. She was in too much pain to bond with her baby for the first three weeks of its life. There are many more stories, some even more tragic.

We at ACOG believe that it is unrealistic to exclude the mother and provide services solely to the fetus. It is impossible to separate mother-baby pairs and expect a good outcome for either of them.

WOMEN AT RISK WILL THERE BE COVERAGE?

According to the Centers for Disease Control and Prevention (CDC), "each day in the United States, two to three women die of pregnancy complications." The CDC further notes that "childbirth remains the most common reason for hospitalization in the United States, and pregnancies with complications result in more costly hospitalization." Half of all maternal deaths in this country might be prevented through early diagnosis and appropriate medical care of pregnancy complications.

African American women, Hispanic women who have immigrated to the United States, and American Indian and Alaska Native women are at greatest risk for maternal mortality. CDC statistics note that African American women are four times as likely to die of pregnancy complications compared with white women, and American Indian and Alaska Native women are nearly twice as likely to die. In a 14-year national study of pregnancy-related deaths in the United States, CDC found that the pregnancy-related mortality ratio for African American women was 25.1 deaths per 100,000 live births, and Hispanic women was 10.3 deaths per 100,000 live births, versus 6.0 per 100,000 deaths for non-Hispanic white women. Poverty and lack of insurance certainly play a significant role in these alarming statistics.

The Administration is right to target prenatal coverage to reduce these figures. For many women, especially minority women, however, complications also arise after giving birth. And the truth is, postpartum women without health insurance are more likely to go without care because of economic priorities. The other truth is, sick women who recently delivered are less able to care for their babies. In this way, a lack of postpartum care harms mothers and their newborns. The regulation's omission for postpartum coverage will disproportionately affect the very women that need the most help and who experience the highest rate of maternal morbidity and mortality.

As we have stated before, prenatal and intrapartum services are essential. It is inconceivable that there are diseases that affect the mother principally and that have no overall affect on the fetus. Diseases such as diabetes and hypertension clearly have defined fetal effects. Maternal obesity, which requires nutrition counseling, behavioral interventions, and anesthesia consultation is not a health condition limited to the mother. Another patient of mine at 32 weeks pregnant arrived in the emergency room clutching her head with pain and developed confusion over time. A CT scan revealed a large brain tumor. Yes, this is a maternal condition but you can imagine that the effects of neurosurgery and postoperative pain management all had an impact on her developing fetus.

IMPLEMENTATION CONCERNS

Finally, ACOG also has several concerns about the implementation of the Administration's regulation and the impact it will have on ob-gyn practices. Already, the health care system prevents physicians from spending needed time with patients. Skyrocketing medical liability premiums, onerous regulatory paperwork, and continued Medicare payment cuts make everyday practice an endeavor for most physicians. This regulation will create even more bureaucracy and red tape for physicians.

As in the last example, figuring out which components of a patient's care would be covered by such restrictive services would be an impossible task. Because this regulation limits coverage to services directly related to the health of the fetus, ob-gyns will be unsure whether medically necessary care will be covered. In most cases, physicians will simply provide the care and worry after the fact about coverage issues, knowing that a tremendous amount of staff time and effort will be expended to recover even some payment. Furthermore, pregnant women may wonder if they even have the ability to access coverage for non-obstetric conditions or injuries, and decide to simply not seek any treatment. This uncertainty about coverage will discourage physicians from participating and deter women from seeking appropriate, necessary care.

ENACT S. 724

I urge the Senate to quickly pass S. 724 and encourage the Administration to support enactment of this bill to expand coverage to uninsured pregnant women ensuring access to comprehensive prenatal and postpartum coverage. The recently issued regulation, while misdirected in its approach, creates a policy foundation that makes prenatal care and healthy babies a priority. We urge Congress to take the next step and pass S. 724, assuring women's health and their babies healthy lives.

PREPARED STATEMENT OF CRISTINA BEATO, M.D.

Mr. Chairman and Senator Gregg, I want to thank you for accepting our request to include a statement for the record. The Secretary has asked that I serve as the Administration's witness at hearings covering women's health issues of this nature, and the following is my prepared statement.

I would also like to take this opportunity to recognize the members of the Senate Health, Education, Labor and Pensions Committee for their continued interest in addressing the needs of low-income pregnant women and their children. Like their colleagues on the Finance Committee, they have demonstrated a clear concern that women and children receive the best this country can offer in the way of health care, and we think they should be commended for that.

As Congress and this committee seek input and explore ways to address the lack of insurance for many pregnant women, I want to re-emphasize HHS' commitment to implement policies that will provide more women coverage for a healthy pregnancy and safe delivery. The health of pregnant women and a healthy start for their children is certainly a goal we all share and that we are all working toward in our respective roles in government. I want to give some examples of some of the avenues we are exploring through administrative authority.

Current law gives HHS the authority to provide prenatal and delivery care to many low-income pregnant mothers and their unborn children. The Secretary has exercised that authority and, after conducting a thorough regulatory process, including a public comment period, a final rule has been published that will allow states to extend S-CHIP coverage to unborn children and their mothers. The rule will ensure that pregnant women and children who are currently ineligible for health care under either Medicaid or S-CHIP are given the support they need for a healthy pregnancy and delivery. All children deserve a healthy start in life, and this rule is one more option states have to fulfill that promise to low-income mothers and babies.

Under the regulation, we are able to reach a broad population of vulnerable women and children because we can offer coverage to the children of immigrants who are otherwise ineligible for any coverage. The legislative proposal S. 724 would not reach this broader population of low-income women and children.

A point of consistency across the legislative proposals and the Administration policy is that the benefits, and hence services covered, (prenatal and pregnancy related services) are the same, excluding postpartum care after hospitalization. While eligibility for these benefits extends through the child rather than the mother under the rule, the benefits and services covered remain the same. The concern that mothers would not receive care while still hospitalized immediately following delivery is addressed in the published rule's comment and response section, and has again been addressed in correspondence with Congress and in discussions with key stakeholders in the effort to improve the health of mothers and children.

The regulation also affords states the opportunity to access enhanced-match funds without conditioning this access on any eligibility expansions at the regular match rate. Again, the pending legislative proposals would condition access to enhanced-match funds for some states. And, since states already have the option to raise eligibility at their regular match rate and have not chosen to do so, we believe the regulation provides them the opportunity to cover more low-income pregnant women.

In fact, President Bush's fiscal year 2003 budget proposed to strengthen the SCHIP program by making available to states unused SCHIP funds that otherwise would return to the federal treasury. The SCHIP law originally required that states that did not use their full SCHIP allotment during the previous three years return the unused funds. Under the President's plan, these unused funds would be made available for states nationwide to expand coverage to the uninsured, especially those at the lowest end of the income scale. Congress can be a partner in this initiative by enacting at least this component of the Administration's budget.

Adopting the President's proposal on unused SCHIP funds would not only complement this new rule, but many of the other initiatives in the Administration's larger effort to give mothers and children a healthy start and help those who cannot afford health insurance get the health care that they need. Already, the Administration has made unprecedented strides in assisting states to expand health care services.

Since January 2001, HHS has approved waivers and plan amendments that have expanded eligibility to more than 2 million people and enhanced services for 6 million Americans. In August 2001, Secretary Thompson launched the Health Insurance Flexibility and Accountability (HIFA) Initiative to encourage states to expand access to health care coverage for low-income individuals through Medicaid and SCHIP demonstrations. The initiative gives states more flexibility to coordinate these companion programs and offers simplified applications for states that commit to reducing the number of people without health insurance. Seven states have approved HIFA waivers: New Mexico, California, Arizona, Maine, Illinois, Colorado and Oregon.

For example, New Mexico's HIFA demonstration will cover uninsured parents of Medicaid and SCHIP children, as well as childless adults, in partnership with employers in the State. Up to 40,000 currently uninsured individuals may be covered under the demonstration with a projected implementation date of February 2003. This waiver includes coverage for prenatal care, labor and delivery and postpartum care. California's HIFA waiver will cover up to 275,000 parents, relative caretakers and legal guardians. Arizona expects to expand coverage for up to 48,000, and Illinois expects 300,000 additional parents will be covered. Colorado's HIFA demonstration expands coverage to 13,000 uninsured pregnant women. In addition, through the Administration's Pharmacy Plus Model Waiver Initiative, states are able to expand drug coverage to low-income seniors and people with disabilities. Five Pharmacy Plus waivers Florida, Illinois, Maryland, South Carolina and Wisconsin have been approved so far.

Again, while waivers often result in the expansion of coverage for health benefits and services, the Administration also has programs that help communities provide health services to low-income women directly, including prenatal and pregnancy related care. Most of these services are administered by the Health Resources and Services Administration (HRSA) and, in particular, the Maternal and Child Health Bureau (MCHB). Programs supported through Title V of the Social Security Act (the MCH Block Grant) provide gap-filling prenatal health services to more than 2 million women each year.

In addition, in FY2001, the Healthy Start program funded 106 grants to communities with a total of $90 million to improve perinatal health and improve prenatal care among at-risk populations. In FY2002, Healthy Start was able to extend services further by funding an additional 12 sites in high-risk communities, expanding outreach, case-management, and preventive health services.

The MCHB has also begun new programs focusing on reducing risk factors for adverse outcomes during pregnancy, especially among vulnerable women. This includes screening for tobacco use, domestic violence, alcohol use, depression, and substance abuse then referring as needed.

HRSA-supported Community Health Centers serve more than 3 million women of childbearing age and provide primary care services, including prenatal, delivery, and postpartum care, for low-income women who are likely to lack access to health insurance or other sources of care. Funding for Community Health Centers has been increased substantially under a five-year expansion plan initiated by President Bush.

I hope this brief overview highlighting just some of the initiatives this Administration has implemented and supported provides a more comprehensive view of our commitment to improving the health of low-income women and children. I believe that while undertaking a balanced dialogue and delving into the substance of both the problems that result when women and children lack access to health care and current and proposed solutions, we should never lose sight of our shared goal. On behalf of HHS, I hope that we can work together with the many organizations that share our vision of a healthier beginning for children to encourage states to expand coverage under SCHIP to unborn children and their mothers.

There is still work to be done to meet our universal goal of giving children a healthy start in life, and we look forward to continued collaboration with Congress.

Prepared Statement of Lisa Bernstein

Mr. Chairman, members of the committee, I am honored to come before you today to urge passage of S.724, the "Mothers and Newborns Health Insurance Act of 2001."

First, I would like to tell you how I have come to be here and a bit about why The What To Expect Foundation was formed.

The What To Expect Foundation takes its name from the bestselling What To Expect pregnancy and parenting series that was written by the Foundation's president, Heidi Murkoff and her mother, the late Arlene Eisenberg.

This series of books has helped over 20 million families from pregnancy through their child's toddler years. What To Expect When You're Expecting is often referred to as "America's Pregnancy Bible." According to a USA TODAY poll it is read by 93% of all mothers that buy a pregnancy guide the What To Expect series of books are not only the three bestselling parenting books in the country—they are among the bestselling books in the country on any topic This week What To Expect When You're Expecting is #3 on the New York Times bestseller list.

But I'm sorry to say, as many parents as the What To Expect books have helped, they've missed many more. As you know, our nation's infant mortality rate is higher than 28 other countries; we're right behind Cuba. And even if a mother could afford to buy a prenatal guide she might not be able to read it. The literacy rate in the United States is a continuing problem. Today 21% to 23% of adults—or some 40 to 44 million people across the country read at less than a fifth grade level.

Thus the birth of The What To Expect Foundation a non-profit organization dedicated to helping mothers in-need receive prenatal health and literacy education so they too can expect healthy pregnancies, safe deliveries and—can read to their babies.

The BABY BASICS program provides prenatal education that takes into account the special health, economic, social and cultural needs of low-income women and gives prenatal providers culturally appropriate health literacy tools and support.

By 2003 we will have provided over 200,000 women with the BABY BASICS program in English and Spanish we are now building model BABY BASICS health literacy sites at clinics across the country.

While researching the BABY BASICS book and program I had the opportunity to speak to hundreds of pregnant, low-income women, and the doctors, midwives, nurses, outreach workers, educators and social workers that care for them.

From across the country I heard the pregnancy stories of our country's poorest women some were stories about swollen feet, indigestion, back pain. Others were about hopes and fears that cut across income and education—will I be a good mother, will I know how to hold a child? Will I be able to provide for my baby?

But too many of these stories broke my heart. Teens who were pregnant because they wanted someone to love and to love them, women, pregnant with no health insurance, who work long days for little income, and had to take off unpaid time to sit in a hard chair for hours waiting for an unscheduled 5 minute free appointment at a crowded clinic. Women who saw a doctor for the first time the day their water broke- because they could not afford care.

Secretary Thompson did an important thing and is to be congratulated when he realized that many pregnant women could not afford prenatal care. One look at the infant mortality rate, and he looked for ways to fix it. He also realized that SCHP a dramatically successful program for families had the funds and the ability to reach out to help in our constant battle against infant and maternal mortality. And I applaud him for finding a stop-gap measure that was within his domain to help states provide pre-natal care quickly and efficiently by extending the care to the fetus with an implicit understanding that this was a quick-fix, one that would be remedied by legislation.

Now, frankly, I'm confused. In his recent letters to you, Senators, he seems to have changed his mind, saying such legislation is no longer needed. His quick fix is enough.

But the quick fix put forward by the administration is not really a fix at all. Because now we've created even more problems after we're spent so much time and money promoting pre-natal care we've gone and created an entirely new funded medical program—called "fetal care".

Because "fetal care" and "prenatal care" are not the same thing. Please, let me tell you why.

Pre-natal care is about dignity. Fetal care is about shame.

This September, Secretary Thompson, Senator Kennedy, and Senator Hatch, along with our Foundation's president, Heidi Murkoff, spoke at Robert Wood Johnson's Covering Kids celebration, that honored SCHP's 5th anniversary. Mothers and fathers explained how Child Health Plus helped their family. These were working families, with two jobs, working double-shifts to keep their families afloat.

One family, suddenly unemployed, had no idea how they were going to pay for their daughter's continuing diabetes care until they found SCHP. Another hard working mother spoke about SCHP paying for surgery that saved her boy's life.

These parents were heroes to their children, and to the audience. With the help of SCHP they had provided for their families. Because SCHP has been carefully crafted, marketed and promoted as help for working families and children these parents were able to retain their dignity, and were proud of their ability, as parents, to provide the health care their child needed, when they needed it.

Just as offering pre-natal care to a woman can help her afford to do the best for her unborn child. Its friendly help, that is offered with dignity and can be accepted with pride.

Offering "fetal care" is a slap in the face. This new regulation makes clear that fetal care is about the fetus first. "Extras" like epidurals and pain medication will only be available if a case can be made that they are for the health of the fetus. Fetal care offers the mother no dignity, devaluing her life which she risks by sharing her body with the unborn child.

Pre-natal care acknowledges that there are two things that grow when a woman becomes pregnant. First, of course, there's the fetus, growing to become a healthy baby. And second, and no less importantly, there's the woman who also must grow she must grow to think of herself as a mother a parent, a provider. Inextricably linked in a dance as old as creation mother and child grow together—both nurtured with love and care.

"Fetal care" unbinds those ties—breaks those bonds. It's about the government choosing fetuses over women, providing the fetus will all of its health care needs while saying to the woman we can't help you.

Pre-natal care provides a woman with the comprehensive health coverage she needs to have a baby. It cares for her body and her health. It helps her stay strong so she can be strong as a mother. It provides for her needs before and after the delivery, and gives her the chance to recover so she has the strength and the health to nurse her precious new bundle.

"Fetal care" tells mothers that once they've had the baby they're on their own. Like Cinderella after the ball, once the baby is delivered, no more fairy godmother. Suddenly her health care is gone. No glass slipper. Even her 48 hours guaranteed hospital stay is out of the picture.

Pre-natal care is about family values. It helps create parents. It does what Early Head Start, Head Start, Healthy Start and Even Start do so well it gives parents the strong shoulders they need to make sure no child is left behind. It fosters optimism.

"Fetal care" throws the parent out with the bathwater. It fosters pessimism, and an early pervading sense of failure. From the start it fails to acknowledge that a parent is a child's first and best teacher. To me, "fetal care" fosters foster-care.

Pre-natal care fills hospital wards with healthy babies.

Fetal care fills hospitals with wards of the state.

Senators, so many good things can happen when a women gets proper, comprehensive pre-natal care. As you've heard, The What To Expect Foundation links prenatal care to literacy training. So women learn how to read, and learn how to read to their babies. Healthy Start and other programs across the country are linking prenatal care to all kinds of positive, self-esteem building social programs. Parenting skills, job training, long-term housing planning, financial planning.

We have trouble getting women into pre-natal care why would we ever want to put up any barriers to pre-natal care? Secretary Thompson has done an honorable thing by opening the door to pre-natal care for thousands of women each year. But imaginary barriers, liberal barriers, conservative barriers, unintended barriers? No matter what we want to call these barriers regardless of their politics or their intent, they are unnecessary barriers to care. I'm here to tell you that hundreds of providers, practically every doctor, midwife and nurse across the country agrees that this fetal care quick-fix must not stand as a barrier. And every mother including this mother and the mothers who have told millions of mothers across the country What To Expect agree—Our job is to knock down the barriers. Passing S724 will remove those barriers.

And then we can roll up our sleeves and get back to work. Because only a healthy parent can provide a healthy future for a healthy child.

Prepared Statement of Kate Michelman

NARAL applauds the Committee for holding this hearing to highlight the current lack of adequate health-care coverage for pregnant women and children, and explore potential solutions.

NARAL's mission is to guarantee every woman the right to make personal decisions regarding the full range of reproductive choices, including preventing unintended pregnancy, bearing healthy children, and choosing legal abortion. NARAL has 26 affiliates nationwide and nearly 300,000 members and supporters. On behalf of our membership and pro-choice Americans, NARAL submits this testimony to: (1) illuminate what is at stake for reproductive rights by making embryos, not women, beneficiaries of governmental health care programs and provide context illustrating the dangers inherent in the Administration's chosen course; and (2) advocate for greater coverage of pregnant women under SCHIP's existing framework or new legislation such as that sponsored by Senator Bingaman.

The Stakes and The Context. A woman's right to choose is in peril, jeopardized by a fragile consensus on the part of the Supreme Court in favor of legal abortion and an Administration determined to make use of every power at its disposal to roll back women's reproductive freedom.

Up to now, the Bush Administration has been pursuing an incremental campaign to denigrate and restrict a woman's right to choose. We have seen the nomination of anti-choice judges for the federal district and appellate courts, support for anti-choice legislation such as the Child Custody Protection Act and the Unborn Victims of Violence Act, Executive Orders attacking the reproductive rights of women around the world, appointment of anti-choice officials to key cabinet and sub-cabinet positions, statements of support for groups seeking the overturn of Roe v. Wade, and the filing of a legal brief supporting restrictions on a woman's freedom to choose. Dr. W. David Hager, strongly credentialed in anti-choice activism, is the rumored favorite to head the Food and Drug Administration's Reproductive Health Drugs Advisory Committee. Health agencies from the Centers for Disease Control and Prevention to the National Institutes of Health have begun censoring their websites for material offensive to the ideology of the hard right that is, material disproving anti-choice propaganda about abortion, sex education, sexually transmitted diseases, and HIV prevention.

Against this backdrop, this month the Administration took a significant step towards its ultimate goal of making abortion illegal. On October 3, 2002, the Bush Administration published a final rule that would actually designate embryos and fetuses as "children" eligible for medical benefits independent of the pregnant woman under the State Children's Health Insurance Program (SCHIP) (42 C.F.R. 457 (2002)). Under the joint federal/state SCHIP program, states provide health care to low-income children who are not covered by the Medicaid program. The Administration took this unorthodox course, notwithstanding the fact that both SCHIP and Medicaid law allow states to cover more pregnant women than would otherwise be eligible under the state's income limits to ensure quality prenatal care.

Although the rule on its face does not change the status of legal abortion, any challenge to Roe v. Wade that reaches the Supreme Court will surely contend that an evolving legal trend recognizes fetuses as persons. In support of this contention, opponents of Roe will point to state legislation recognizing embryos and fetuses as persons in a variety of circumstances, and this new SCHIP rule will be an essential piece of evidence for their argument. The Administration's interim strategy to prepare the way for a challenge to Roe is underway. To protect the foundation of Roe v. Wade, NARAL thus opposes this rule that distinguishes the embryo's or fetus' interests from those of the pregnant woman.

In a more immediate sense, the new rule could actually do harm to women by pitting them against the program's "patients" the embryos. Under this regulation, would a pregnant woman with cancer be able to access potentially life-saving radiation treatment or chemotherapy, since such treatment could harm the embryo? The effects of many prescription drugs on pregnancies have not been studied; under this rule, a woman's treatment for any variety of medical conditions might be denied, in favor of the embryo or fetus. If a woman were carrying an embryo or fetus covered under this new proposal and she had a miscarriage, there would no longer be a "beneficiary" for the SCHIP program. Would the government then refuse to pay for her follow-up care?

It is commonly understood as a matter of public health that healthy women tend to have healthier babies, and as a legal matter that the woman should make all decisions relating to her pregnancy. The rule imposes a new paradigm separating the woman from her pregnancy, and allowing a government health care program to work on behalf of the fetus, without any reference to the woman herself. That is, the new rule would not provide care for the woman only care for the fetus. A woman's pre-existing conditions, such as diabetes or asthma, could apparently only be treated if and to the extent that such treatment would benefit the fetus. Doctors might well face confusion about basic preventive or maintenance care for the woman would her medical conditions only be covered when they worsened so as to jeopardize the pregnancy? As a practical matter, then, this rule is either unworkable or unethical, in setting up potential conflicts between the woman's interests and fetal interests.

In an unexpected move, the Administration's rule also allows the embryos and fetuses of immigrant pregnant women to be covered under SCHIP. This creates a strange dichotomy because under current law, legal immigrants cannot receive Medicaid or SCHIP benefits until they have been in the country for five years. (Illegal immigrants do not qualify at all.) As a legal matter, the regulation treats immigrant pregnant women as if their embryos and fetuses were already born here as citizens and were thus entitled to the full benefits of citizenry. As a practical effect of this expanded concept of citizenship, the three year-old daughter of a recently immigrated pregnant woman cannot receive publicly funded health care, but the woman's fetus can. This illustrates that the true nature of this rule is not to deliver health care to children who need it for the three year old surely needs care but to grant fetuses special legal rights.

In sum, the Administration's failure to address the many practical problems with implementing this rule problems NARAL identified in our comments opposing the proposed rule indicates that its SCHIP regulation is not serious health-care policy; instead, it is a political statement and a legal stratagem.

An alternative vision. NARAL has long supported initiatives to provide prenatal care for pregnant women; indeed, the millions of uninsured deserve comprehensive health care. Women planning pregnancy and the children they bear benefit immensely from high-quality care, and conversely, the chronic lack of access to a continuum of services for low-income women jeopardizes the promise of healthy pregnancies and healthy childbearing.

For many months, the Administration tried to play expanded health care coverage both ways: it said it supported legislation expanding SCHIP eligibility, while at the same time issuing the proposed (now final) rule making embryos and fetuses federal health care beneficiaries. The other shoe has now dropped. The Administration's recent reversal, announcing that it no longer supports legislation expanding SCHIP to cover pregnant women, must be met with determined Congressional opposition. The Administration's about-face reveals that its real goal is a legal and political one endowing fetuses with legal rights and shoring up its ideological base rather than a substantive policy goal. Moreover, as a matter of separation of powers and the proper allocation of governmental responsibilities, the regulation is a significant policy change, one that should be overridden by Congress.

NARAL urges Congress to enact legislation allowing states to expand their SCHIP programs to pregnant women, which would effectively nullify the regulation. The best way to assure healthy pregnancies and healthy childbearing is to provide dependable, quality care for pregnant women, and NARAL commends Senator Bingaman and others for their efforts in this connection and continues to urge Congress' passage of legislation that does so.

Congress must set the legal and political record straight: pregnant women deserve health care coverage. Governmental agencies entrusted to protect the public health cannot be misused as vehicles for advancing an anti-choice political agenda to the detriment of Americans' health.

Prepared Statement of Priscilla Smith

The Center for Reproductive Law and Policy (CRLP) commends the Committee for underscoring the rights of pregnant women to safe pregnancy through this hearing and through the "Mothers and Newborns Health Insurance Act" (S. 724). CRLP is a non-profit legal advocacy organization dedicated to protecting and defending women's reproductive rights, including the rights of pregnant women to safe pregnancy. CRLP submits this testimony to support efforts to expand access to pregnancy-related care through legislation such as the "Mothers and Newborns Health Insurance Act." This bill not only addresses a significant gap in our nation's healthcare system, but also mitigates the negative effects of misguided amendments to the State Children's Health Insurance Program (SCHIP) recently adopted by the Department of Health and Human Services.

I. "Mothers and Newborns Health Insurance Act" Addresses a Significant Healthcare Gap

Currently, the United States ranks twenty-first in the world in rates of maternal mortality and twenty-eighth in the world in rates of infant mortality. It is estimated that every week, 8,500 children in the United States are born to mothers who lack access to prenatal care. Furthermore, it is likely that half of all maternal deaths in the United States could be prevented through early diagnosis and appropriate medical treatment of pregnancy complications. This is shocking given the availability of unsurpassed medical care and technology in the United States and widespread knowledge of the importance of early and ongoing prenatal care to help ensure a healthy pregnancy and optimal birth outcome.

A primary barrier to timely prenatal care, and thus to improving the health of pregnant women and newborns in the United States, is a lack of health insurance coverage. Despite the Medicaid expansions implemented in the late 1980s and early 1990s, recently released figures from the March of Dimes indicated that nearly one in five women of childbearing age (ages 15-44 years) in the United States were still uninsured in 1999. See Kenneth E. Thorpe et al., The Distribution of Health Insurance Coverage Among Pregnant Women, 1999, prepared for the March of Dimes (Apr. 2001), available at http://www.modimes.org/files/2001FinalThorpeReport.pdf (last visited Apr. 16, 2002). Thus, further expansions are necessary to reach the uninsured.

Moreover, as this Committee and the Administration have recognized, there is a troubling disparity in access to prenatal care between white women and minority women. Rates of maternal mortality and morbidity and infant mortality which are highest among non-white populations reflect this disparity. While research suggests that racial and ethnic inequalities in medical treatment would persist in some measure even if access to health insurance were equalized, see Key Facts: Race, Ethnicity, and Medical Care, The Henry J. Kaiser Family Foundation (October 1999), it also appears that increased access to health insurance coverage would reduce these disparities based on race and ethnicity. Id.

Therefore, increasing access to health insurance coverage for pregnant women is vital for two reasons. First, insuring access to early and ongoing pregnancy-related care for women in all ethnic and racial groups must be the first step in any efforts to reduce overall rates of maternal mortality and morbidity, and to erase the disparity between the quality of care received by women of color and white women. Second, increased access to prenatal care will improve the health of newborns throughout the country and similarly work to erase disparities in infant mortality rates between racial and ethnic groups.

The "Mothers and Newborns Health Insurance Act" serves these goals by increasing access to insurance coverage. The legislation provides insurance coverage for prenatal care, delivery and post-partum care to targeted, low-income pregnant women. The legislation also provides coverage for newborns for their first year of life. Through these provisions, S. 724 ensures better birth outcomes and healthier mothers and children.

II. THE "MOTHERS AND NEWBORNS HEALTH INSURANCE ACT" IS FAR SUPERIOR TO THE NEW SCHIP REGULATION AMENDMENTS.

Unlike S. 724, the recent amendments to the State Children's Health Insurance Program (SCHIP), promulgated by the Department of Health and Human Services (HHS), fail to adequately address the overwhelming need for healthcare coverage for pregnant women. Instead of extending benefits to pregnant women, the new regulation classifies the fetus as an "unborn child" and expands coverage to "an individual in the period between conception and birth up to age 19." 67 FR 61956-01 (Oct. 2, 2002). It is greatly disturbing that HHS has promoted amendments to the SCHIP regulations to extend the plan to cover fetuses, while patently ignoring the health needs of pregnant women. This new policy is fraught with legal and practical problems:

The regulation could place the health of pregnant women at risk and threatens a woman's integral right to control her own healthcare.

By defining a fetus as a "child" from the moment of conception for purposes of SCHIP, the regulation is in clear tension with fundamental principles of constitutional law.

Low-income pregnant women deserve actual, not merely incidental, health insurance coverage that covers all of their pregnancy-related needs.

There are superior means of ensuring prenatal care for women whose incomes fall within the SCHIP-eligibility criteria in their state, such as the "Mothers and Newborns Health Insurance Act."

CRLP has significant concerns with the new amendments, as outlined below. CRLP urges Congress to enact the "Mothers and Newborns Health Insurance Act" to address and remedy the significant gaps left by the SCHIP program.

A. By Covering the Zygote, Embryo or Fetus and Not the Woman Herself, the Regulation Could Place the Health of Pregnant Women at Risk.

Although the Administration claims that the goal of the new regulation is to provide for comprehensive prenatal care in order to improve the pregnant woman's health, the mechanism chosen could actually place the woman herself at risk. The regulation does not provide any insurance coverage for pregnant women in the post-partum period, nor does it provide for comprehensive care for pregnant women during either pregnancy, or labor and delivery.

First, the standard of care for pregnant women requires continuity of medical treatment from prenatal care through post-partum care. The American College of Obstetricians and Gynecologists (ACOG) and the American Academy of Pediatrics (AAP) recommend that the physical and psychosocial status of the mother be assessed on an ongoing basis following hospital discharge. They further recommend that four to six weeks after delivery the mother should receive a post-partum review and examination. American Academy of Pediatrics & American College of Obstetricians and Gynecologists, Guidelines for Perinatal Care (4th ed. 1997).

Unfortunately, the regulation does not allow states to provide SCHIP coverage to pregnant women for any post-partum care. This is because under the regulation, SCHIP would cover only the "child" in utero, not the pregnant woman. While the pregnant woman would incidentally receive some covered care as a result of carrying the "child" within her uterus, that covered care would be available only during "the period from conception to birth." The moment after the birth of her child, a woman who may have been covered for any incidental care as a result of having an SCHIP-covered fetus in utero, would appear to lose insurance coverage. The woman would therefore not be eligible for any covered care during the post-partum period, including for the post-delivery hospital stay, care for her incision received during a Cesarean section delivery, for an episiotomy or any other post-delivery complications. This result flies in the face of sound medical and public health policy, not to mention the regulation's stated goals.

In contrast, S. 724 provides coverage to pregnant women for post-partum care, thus remedying this troubling omission.

Second, by insuring only the fetus, it is unclear whether the regulation authorizes insurance coverage for pregnant women for medical treatments that do not have a direct impact on the well-being of the fetus. Thus, for example, if an epidural is needed during delivery, would that be covered even though it would benefit only the woman, and not the fetus? If the woman broke her leg during the pregnancy, would treatment be covered? And, since eligibility for benefits only exists in relation to a living fetus, it is unclear whether any benefits would be available to the mother for complications following a miscarriage technically, since the beneficiary is no longer alive, such benefits would not be available. While we agree with the statement made by Secretary Thompson regarding the importance of prenatal services as "a vital, life-long determinant of health" for the fetus, HHS to Allow States to Provide SCHIP Coverage for Prenatal Care, HHS News Release, January 31, 2002, we believe that ensuring meaningful health benefits for the pregnant woman is an equally important goal, and one that this regulation fails to meet but that S. 724 directly addresses.

Third, targeting coverage to the fetus also appears to create serious conflicts over health care decision making, all of which threaten a woman's integral right to control her own healthcare. It is unclear under the regulation how the interests of the fetus and the pregnant woman should be balanced when their health care needs diverge, or where treatments needed by the pregnant woman could actually be harmful to the fetus. For example, a woman with mental illness may require medications, such as lithium, that are contraindicated for the fetus. See, e.g., Jennifer R. Niebyl, M.D., Drugs in Pregnancy and Lactation, in Steven G. Gabbe, M.D., Jennifer R. Niebyl, M.D., Joe Leigh Simpson, M.D., eds., Obstetrics: Normal and Problem Pregnancies at 249, 255 (3d ed. 1996). Similarly, a woman diagnosed with breast cancer may not be covered for radiation treatments needed to save her life. Would the treatments in these cases be covered? Could the state intervene on behalf of the fetus? What would happen if the life-saving treatment was for the fetus, but it endangered the mother could the mother be compelled to undergo the treatment? Who would decide these types of coverage questions the state, the federal government, the doctor, or the pregnant woman herself? Could the state or the other parent's health care decisions trump the pregnant woman's, even where her own health could be adversely affected? These are all troubling questions that are raised by the regulation but that would not be implicated by S. 724 since the legislation recognizes the pregnant woman's right to healthcare.

B. This Regulation Seeks to Chip Away at Fundamental Principles of Constitutional Law.

By defining a fetus as a "child" from the moment of conception for purposes of SCHIP, the regulation is in clear tension with fundamental principles of constitutional law. The Supreme Court clearly stated in Roe v. Wade that "[T]he word 'person,' as used in the Fourteenth Amendment, does not include the unborn," 410 U.S. 113,158 (1973). The Administration's impractical attempt to force the definition of a child to include a fetus results in bizarre outcomes and administrative confusion, revealing the Administration's true goal of chipping away at fundamental rights. For instance, under current law, states track eligibility for public benefits using Social Security numbers, which all Americans receive when they are born. Since fetuses are not eligible for Social Security numbers, it is unclear how states will track their eligibility for benefits until they are born. Will they create a whole new individual identifier just for fetuses? There will be further implications for tax rules as well. Generally, an American citizen is only counted for taxation purposes after they are born. Does the granting of legal personhood under the regulation mean that fetuses could be taxed inside the womb? Alternatively, could they be claimed as a deduction before they are born? These examples demonstrate the irrationality of this policy and the confusing results it would generate.

Other Supreme Court cases, such as Planned Parenthood of Southeastern Pennsylvania v. Casey, 505 U.S. 833 (1992) and Stenberg v. Carhart, 530 U.S. 914 (2000) have emphasized the importance of protecting women's health in the face of laws restricting access to abortion. Because the regulation elevates the fetus' health to the potential detriment of the woman's health, this conflict places the regulation in further tension with Supreme Court precedent by potentially jeopardizing the woman's health.

The regulation indicates that the Administration cares more about promoting the "rights" of a fertilized egg with an eye to building the legal foundation to overturn the Supreme Court decision in Roe v. Wade, than it does about women's health. The best way to improve women's health is to recognize their right and ability to make private, medical decisions about their own bodies.

C. The Regulation Denigrates Women Without Achieving Its Purported Goal.

Low-income pregnant women deserve actual, not merely incidental, health insurance coverage that covers all of their pregnancy-related needs, including those that extend into the critical post-partum period. By providing insurance for the fertilized egg or fetus, but not for the woman herself, this regulation denigrates women treating them as mere vessels for a fetus, undeserving of health care in their own right. Given the superiority of these alternative means of achieving improved birth outcomes (see below), the Administration's decision to promulgate the regulation—and inexplicably withdraw support for other measures—must be seen as a political gambit, unrelated to improved pregnancy-related care. It can only be seen as an ideologically-based attempt to redefine a fetus as a "person," in conflict with the Supreme Court's ruling in Roe v. Wade, 410 U.S. 113 (1973) without regard to whether health care coverage is actually increased.

D. There Are Superior Means of Ensuring Prenatal Care for Women Whose Incomes Fall Within the SCHIP-Eligibility Criteria in Their State, Including the "Mothers and Newborns Health Insurance Act."

The regulation is all the more unacceptable because it is not necessary to ensure prenatal care for women whose incomes fall within the SCHIP-eligibility criteria in their state. There are at least two superior means of achieving this goal: 1) the "Mothers and Newborns Health Insurance Act," which has been proposed with bipartisan support to expand SCHIP to include pregnant women; and, 2) until federal legislation is in place, a streamlined process for obtaining §1115 waivers to add pregnant women to a state's SCHIP program (as New Jersey and Rhode Island have done).

CRLP supports the regulation's stated goal of expanding access to early and regular prenatal care in order to ensure the health of both pregnant women and newborns, but questions SCHIPS' approach of allowing health insurance coverage for a zygote, embryo and fetus in utero. Because there are other less controversial and more effective ways of achieving the stated goal, the Administration's choice of this strategy is curious at best.

V. CONCLUSION

It now falls to Congress to stand up for the healthcare needs of pregnant women through the "Mothers and Newborns Health Insurance Act." CRLP urges the Senate to quickly enact this legislation to expand healthcare coverage to uninsured pregnant women. Once enacted, this legislation would allow states to go beyond the current framework of the SCHIP program and provide insurance to pregnant women in addition to their children.

Thank you.

[Whereupon, at 11:47 a.m., the subcommittee was adjourned.]

○